BRAIN IN A JAR

BRAIN IN A JAR

*A Daughter's Journey through
Her Father's Memory*

Nancy Stearns Bercaw

April 4, 2013

*Barbara,
It's the heart
that belongs in
a jar.
Love,
Nancy*

BROADSTONE

Library of Congress Control Number: 2013931080

ISBN 978-1-937968-05-2

DESIGN AND TYPESETTING BY JONATHAN GREENE

Broadstone Books
An Imprint of Broadstone Media LLC
418 Ann Street
Frankfort, KY 40601-1929
BroadstoneBooks.com

for Beauregard Lee &
David Beauregard

CONTENTS

III. The Ending

We are linked by blood, and blood is memory without language.

—JOYCE CAROL OATES

INTRODUCTION

Alzheimer's knows no party line or national borders. The disease strikes all its victims with the same unrelenting results. Even though people are living longer than ever before, almost half who reach eighty-five years of age will suffer from Alzheimer's. The taxpayer cost of the disease is already more than a hundred billion dollars each year. But the non-taxpayer cost to families is even greater. That's why we joined forces to co-chair the bipartisan Alzheimer's Study Group to make this mounting global epidemic a priority for research and legislation. But even more telling than the statistics of this rising crisis are the stories of the real people who are suffering.

In that vein, we'd like to introduce *Brain in a Jar,* the gut-wrenching tale of a pioneer in the fight against Alzheimer's disease. A man who believed from a very young age that Alzheimer's was a shotgun pointed at the heads of people he loved—and, indeed, his own.

Dr. Beauregard Lee Bercaw, a true American patriot and world citizen, became a neurologist after watching his father—a lawyer who worked for General Douglas MacArthur in pre-war Manila—deteriorate and die from Alzheimer's. Horrified by his father's demise, Dr. Bercaw devoted himself to helping others affected by the disease. As a reminder of this solemn vow and his own genetic predisposition, Dr. Bercaw kept an atrophied brain in a jar on his office desk.

Dr. Bercaw was painfully aware that a cure for Alzheimer's might not be found in his lifetime. Still, he fought the disease—in his patients and in himself—like the Air Force captain he had been during the Vietnam War. When he turned sixty, Dr. Bercaw launched a strategic effort to thwart what he saw as his own impending memory loss. Dr. Bercaw tried everything to buy more time. He also turned his attention to his daughter, Nancy Stearns Bercaw, believing that their strong resemblance meant she was doomed too.

When Dr. Bercaw's valiant battle proved insurmountable, he was moved to a memory care facility in Naples, Florida. And his daughter turned his cause into her own. *Brain in a Jar* is more of a mission than a memoir. Nancy's stories about her father's impassioned life have already garnered great interest and empathy from doctors, families and patients around the world.

Brain in a Jar is an American Gothic tale of love, grief, genetics, obsession, adventure, fear and courage. The Bercaws might break your heart, but they'll also remind you why Alzheimer's disease must take center stage in politics, medicine, and art.

Bob Kerrey and Newt Gingrich

PROLOGUE

After retiring from his neurology practice in Naples, Florida, my father spent hours a day doing math in his head. Even when I was visiting, he would sit silently on his leather recliner with a calculator, verifying the accuracy of his mental arithmetic and his memory of the results. He was trying to stave off what had killed his father. He rarely uttered the name of this disease to me—reserving the phrase "Alzheimer's disease" for clinical use only.

What are you saving your mind for, Dad? I often wondered to myself. *I'm here now, waiting to talk with you.*

On one of these occasions, he suddenly looked up from his Sudoku game and stared at me intensely. I knew it meant that an extreme statement was forthcoming.

"Promise me something, Gal," he said.

"Anything," I answered.

"Swear that you will put a gun to my head if I wind up like my father."

He was dead serious. He collected guns and kept them under lock and key. He knew I could shoot them because he had taught me how.

Before I could speak, he leapt up from his chair.

"Wait. Let me get the family Bible," he said.

My brain was unable to reconcile his request. It wasn't fair or logical to ask a child to kill her own parent. But I knew that fair meant nothing to my father.

In three decades as a neurologist, Dr. Beauregard Lee Bercaw had seen young people die of meningitis faster than their parents could get them to the hospital. He had scooped uncurled gray matter off the emergency room floor hoping to stuff it back in the heads of accident victims. He'd pulled shrapnel out of the skulls of servicemen at Clark Air Base in the Philippines during the Vietnam War.

He came back into the room with the leather-bound King James Bible, which bears the names Nannie Dunlap and Nancy Scott in gold lettering.

"Swear to me," he repeated.

I crossed the fingers on my left hand, just as I had done a hundred times as a kid to protect me from the wrath of lying to my Dad or God. Then, I put my right hand on the Bible.

"I swear," I said, but privately vowed to one day tell the story of the man I couldn't live without.

I

THE BEGINNING

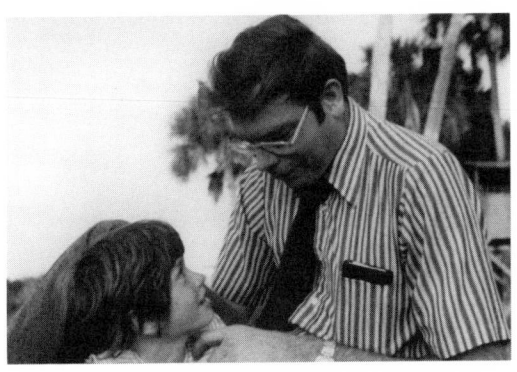

Memory believes before knowing remembers.

—WILLIAM FAULKNER

CHAPTER ONE

THE PUBLIC POOL
HUNTSVILLE, ALABAMA

My father's eyes are fixated on the dozens upon dozens of black folks swimming in Huntsville, Alabama's public pool. It is the summer of 1970. I am five. Beau's face is all scrunched up because he is trying to hide his exasperation. It's the same look he had three years ago when my mother pooped out a 6-foot tapeworm in the Philippines and ran out of our bathroom screaming. I hang on the chain-link fence, gazing at the water and waiting for his frustration to pass. I wish I could look in his ears and see what he's thinking.

"Are we going in, Daddy?" I finally dare to ask.

"Doesn't look like there's much room for us, Gal."

I reach up to grab my father's dangling hand. The pool is full, but since I can't swim yet, we don't need much room, just a spot where my dad can stand and I can hold onto him. He is thirty-two years old, 6 feet 6 inches and 170 pounds. I am tall for my age and scrawny like Beau. This is the way Bercaws are, my father always tells me. We are like this, he says, and we are like that.

"Look! A place!" I yell, pointing to a spot that has just opened up near the rope line separating the shallow and deep ends. "Come on, Daddy, let's go."

We walk in the gates, all eyes on us. It's just like in the Philippines —where I was born five years earlier when Dad was a surgeon at Clark Air Base during the Vietnam War; and where he too, was born when his father worked for General Douglas MacArthur in 1938 Manila.

We Bercaws are white; everyone else is brown and gaping at us. I had overheard my father tell my mother earlier in the morning that we wouldn't be joining the country club where the rich, white folk swam.

"Why not?" she said, with her hands on her slender hips. "All the doctors' wives go there."

"We're not spending money to swim. Water is water."

"I'm not going to a public pool, Beau," my mother said in her sweet lilting voice. She was telling him *and* asking him.

My father courts outsiders. Likewise, the marginalized seek him out. The Huntsville public pool and the bean-pole Bercaws are a match made in heaven.

I take off my skirt and flip-flops and stand by the side of the pool in my bright yellow bathing suit. My dad pulls off his T-shirt that says "University of Virginia." Everyone stops swimming and looks at us, as if their black-and-white television sets had abruptly turned to color. The tallest, pinkest man in Huntsville is about to swim with his five-year-old, blue-eyed, yellow-suited, whiter-than-white, scrawny daughter in a blue-green pool in the heart of black Alabama.

The swimmers fall silent as my father lets himself down the ladder to the open spot. A few people give way slowly, making little ripples. Otherwise, the water is still. No one is moving a muscle. Except for Beau and me.

I walk to the edge and curl my toes over it. I shift my focus to my father, who shoots up among the other swimmers like a bamboo stalk in a rice paddy.

"Jump in, Gal." Beau nods. He looks very serious, the way I think he might when he's about to operate on a patient.

Someone else's father nods at me too, with a big smile on his face. For a second, I wonder if I should jump toward the black man with big white teeth instead of the white man with a big scowl.

I take a big deep breath and exhale loudly, as if I am one of the blue whales that we saw while sailing on the SS *President Cleveland* from the Philippines to California.

The little boy nearest to me starts counting.

"One... two..."

I look back at my dad, whose hands are ready to receive me. Then I inhale.

"Threeeeeeeee!" shrieks the boy.

I leap up as high as I can, kicking my legs while I am still in the air, trying to go higher still. I close my eyes and imagine that I'm flying all the way across the Pacific Ocean. I'm not entirely sure what I will do when I hit the water.

I land in my father's arms, which he's raised above his head to catch me like a pop-fly ball. He lets go and drops me in the water in front of him.

He's teaching me to save my own life. That's the kind of thing he says—words that sound like opposites but actually make sense. Usually, I understand. But when I don't, Beau stares into my eyes and wills me—without words—to figure it out.

Think, Gal, think. I can hear his brain tell mine. Then, once his mind has crept into mine, I hear his next thoughts. *Good, Gal, good.*

When I come up for air, the sound is back on. The waves are splashing again; children are squealing again. I am one of *them* now, not just a part of my father. My chest feels puffed up as big as a life vest. I look at up at Beau, who is grinning big and wide.

He takes a step backward. The people directly behind him scatter.

"Swim," he says.

I do what I had seen the other kids doing when I'd peered through the fence. I kick my feet wildly and paddle my arms while I stare up at him. He never takes his eyes off me.

"Good, Gal. Now put your face down and do it again." He steps back again. Everyone scatters again.

I come up coughing.

"Don't drink it. Blow bubbles." He steps back farther.

Blow, pull, kick, I tell myself. These are the actions that take me to my father. I feel like I am conquering him, as well as the water, with each arrival on his shores.

"Lesson over," he says abruptly. "You can swim."

"Can't we stay?"

"No, it's time to go home."

We pull ourselves out by the ladder and dry off—no one paying us any mind by now. The open spaces we leave behind fill in quickly. It's like we've never been there at all. Except that, in the short time between our arrival and departure, I've learned to swim.

He gives my hand a squeeze when I wave goodbye to the chain-link fence. Beau and I walk home holding hands in silence. I get a pit in my stomach when he's distracted.

"Daddy, can we go back, I want to swim more?" I ask in my sweetest voice.

"Not today, Gal." He squeezes my hand again.

A week later, my father announces it's time for lesson number two. I hadn't known that there would be another. I thought the lesson had been finite. Before it you couldn't swim; after it, you could. The end.

"Put your suit on and get in the car," my father says.

"The car?" I ask. "Why aren't we walking?"

I want to hold his hand and do everything exactly the way we had before.

"Don't ask questions. Just trust."

I lurch into the back seat of our big green Oldsmobile. I sit on my towel to keep the seat from burning me. The window only rolls down partway, so just the top of my head gets a breeze. I watch the houses and shops disappear behind me. Peach and pear trees take their place.

Are palm trees next?

I hope we are going back to the Philippines, even though we had only just moved to Huntsville, Alabama, from Gainesville, Florida, where Dad had been a neurology fellow.

I had asked him then what a neurologist was and he said, "A medical doctor who studies and treats the nervous system." I wanted to say that *he* made me nervous and to ask if he could fix that. But I don't dare because he'll get a weird face. The one that can mean any number of things and it falls on me to figure that out, too. Having a perplexing father is making me smarter. Smart enough to know when not to ask questions.

If Beau and I are going back to the Philippines, I imagine that Mom might want to move in with the country-club people in Huntsville. But I would miss her. She rubbed my back every night and hugged me tight. My mother is as cozy as my father is free. I need them both to keep from getting lost at sea.

Beau interrupts my thoughts. He is thinking about the Philippines too. It's like that with us.

"Gal, did I tell you about the Filipino boy I helped save from being strangulated by a python? You were just a baby then."

"No, how'd ya do it?"

"We taunted the python with a live chicken. I danced that chicken in front of the snake's eyes like the snake charmers I had seen in India. I pretended the chicken was the pendulum of a clock and I tried to hypnotize the python with it. The snake's muscles relaxed and someone grabbed the boy."

"Weren't you scared?"

"Bercaws and Filipinos aren't cowards."

"Are Filipinos scared of Bercaws?"

I'm afraid of my father—not certain which one that made me. I wonder if Beau's father—whom he called Berc—had the same effect on my dad. Berc lives in the Veterans' Hospital in Roanoke because he forgot everything, including his family and himself. I had heard my mom tell someone on the phone that Berc was a mean, nasty man before he lost his mind, and that his ailment might have been a blessing to Beau and his three brothers.

"Everyone's afraid of Bercaws," my dad says from the driver's seat, laughing uproariously. I can see his big blue eyes squinting and watering in the rear-view mirror.

I think of my mother, back at home alone. She plays Go Fish and Candy Land with me for hours, and often lets me win. She says things like, "Oh, Nan! You did it again!" and then bats her blue eyes at me. Beau prefers to bury his head in brain books, but when he does pause to play Checkers with me, he always wins. "Sorry, Gal, you're not good enough to take on your ol' dad."

"Daddy," I yell out from the back seat of our car. "I don't want to go back to the Philippines without Mommy!"

"Don't be a buzzard tail," he says before turning off the main road and onto a dirt one. I pull the towel out from under me and wipe away my tears. I never want him to see his effect on me.

"We're here!"

"Where?"

"The Flint River."

Dad opens my door and goes to get something out of the trunk. I put my bare foot down in the mud. I can see the river down a leafy bank. We had left so quickly that I'd forgotten my flip-flops.

He comes back with a shotgun in his hand. He gets down on one knee and fires up into the trees. I look up to see if any birds fall down. Is he trying to kill a buzzard? I don't dare ask. He'll only tell me things if he feels like it.

"Just scaring the snakes away, that's all, Gal."

"Pythons?"

"Worse. Cottonmouth water moccasins. You're a dead man if one bites you."

"But I'm a little girl, Dad, not a man."

"Then you'll die twice as fast."

I twist up my face. I don't want to be a man or a little girl if either involves being bitten by a snake. Beau will protect me from those slithery rascals, I reckon. But who will protect me from him? I vow to do everything he tells me, and to do it perfectly. Then I will be safe.

Beau puts the gun back in the trunk and lifts me onto his shoulders.

"See that?" he says, pointing to some shiny leaves as he walks to the river. "It's poison ivy. Don't get near it unless you wanna itch for a week."

The ground is a long way down from my father's shoulders, but I can see the leaves he is talking about. I am glad my muddy feet are bouncing against his shirt and not walking on the ground.

"Daddy, did your daddy take you swimming in a river."

I can feel his face scrunch up. He doesn't like this question. I know him.

"No, Gal, my brothers taught me. They threw me into our river and let me sink or swim."

When we get down to the water, my father wades in. I am still on his shoulders. The deepest part goes up to his belly button and touches my toes.

"Stand on my shoulders," he says. "Then jump off and go."

I try to breathe in some of Beau's courage. Then I stand up, holding his hands for support, and propel myself into the air just as I had done off the deck at the public pool. I come up, turn around and try to get back to my father as quickly as possible.

I imagine snakes are chasing me as I swim toward the snake charmer. Kicking and paddling fast takes my mind off the terror. Soon, I forget altogether.

"You're a mermaid," my father says when I get to him, squeezing me tight.

"Even without a tail?" I ask, happy that I have pleased him.

"A slightly deformed one," he laughs. "That's why your ol' dad loves you so much."

My father and I spend the rest of the afternoon playing in those waters. I jump off rocks or tree trunks and swim like crazy to get back into the arms of the only other Filipino Bercaw in the history of the world.

CHAPTER TWO

LYLES BAPTIST CHURCH
PALMYRA, VIRGINIA

I recently turned six. It is 1971. There is a tear coming out of my father's right eye. I watch it move slowly down his cheek until he whisks it away. I wait for another. It doesn't come. I'm sitting sideways so I can watch him.

"Sit straight, Gal," Beau whispers.

My mother, who is on the other side of him, leans over to look at me. She gives me a sweet face. Her black hair is teased up and she has bright red lipstick on her small lips. She is very pale, and I wonder if my mother is actually a ghost—a very beautiful one. She lifts her hand from Beau's knee, and puts her forefinger to her lips to remind me to be quiet and still.

We're outside of Lyles Baptist Church in Palmyra, about seven miles from Rebelanna, the Bercaw family farm. My grandfather is in a coffin being lowered into the ground. A few people are standing around the grave watching him descend. No one is saying anything. The only emotion I see is the solitary tear my father has just produced. If Beau were dead, I would cry my eyes out. Why is there only one tear for Grandfather?

I only saw Berc a few times in my life. He had no idea who I was, but I'd heard a lot about him. Dad told me once that Berc spanked him first thing in the morning to thwart any misbehavior later in the day.

"A preventative whupping," he'd called it. I wasn't sure if my father was telling me as a warning or to tease me. My dad is confusing, but I kinda like that about him. He makes me think. He says Bercaws don't talk unless they have something important to say. I wonder if my dad ever said, "Don't hit me anymore, Father." Surely, that would have been worth breaking the silence.

Even though Berc had been mean to him, Beau worried about his dad when Berc got sick. He had sent Grandmother lots of letters— conveniently from far, far way—about how to take care of Berc.

Clark Air Base, The Philippines 28 May 1967

Berc sounds like he is getting worse + worse. I advise against giving him a lot of pills because they are useless for his condition. Certainly a tranquilizer would be OK to keep him from becoming excessively agitated or worried. You should insist that the druggist label all bottles with the name of the medication– this should always be done anyway because of safety in case of accidental overdosage.

You certainly seem to be managing things well. You must realize, however, it will no longer be possible and that for his own good + your welfare, he will have to be put in a nursing home or an institution.

I have decided to return to Florida for more training in neurology. If I decide to pursue neurosurgery, this will be costly in terms of money, time + inconvenience but I surely would be a better doctor in the long run. If I decide I do not wish to be a neurosurgeon, then it will be the right thing to do anyway.

Nancy + Barbara send their love.

Love,

Beau

My cousin Kathy told me that Berc used to wipe his poop on the yellow wallpaper inside the farmhouse. I looked for traces once, but couldn't find anything other than a squished ant. Kathy is my Uncle David's daughter. They live in Hopewell, near Richmond, just an hour from the farm. She spent a lot more time with Grandmother and Grandfather than I did.

Kathy also said Berc couldn't remember how to get in and out of the tub. Grandmother had put him in a nursing home a few years back, but rescued him when she found out they tied Berc up at night. She brought him back to the farm, and kept him there, until Berc was nothing but a "vegetable," as my dad described him. I imagined Berc as a carrot. He was tall and slim with a jaw that jutted out and big lips on a big mouth—just like my dad and me.

No one ever said what was wrong with Berc, exactly. Memory loss was his "illness." The grown-ups acted like it might be contagious. They said things like, "I wonder if I will get it?"

When Grandmother finally couldn't take care of him one moment longer, Berc was sent to the Veterans' Hospital in Roanoke—per my father's instructions. Berc died alone and confused.

Death by forgetting? It didn't make any sense to me. In fact, it seemed like a nice way to go, especially if you have things in your head that are better off gone.

"It's my fault," Beau told my mother, and I heard him.

If Beau was responsible for Grandfather's brain, am I responsible for his? I thought grownups were supposed to fill up their kids' heads. Maybe the act of raising kids hurts your memory; makes you forget your own life. I vow to be so good that my dad won't ever forget himself. I'll raise myself if necessary.

My grandmother drops some dirt into the grave. She looks regal in a black skirt and jacket and brown pantyhose. She has a black hat pinned to her gray head with a bit of black mesh dangling over her eyes. She has a white hanky in her breast pocket, but she never takes it out. She has a brown mink stole draped over her shoulders.

Uncle Woodson is wearing his military uniform and medals and standing next to her. He is my father's eldest brother and he has three children, including my cousin Nancy Dunlap Bercaw. She is six years older than I am. Her brothers are Woodson and John.

Uncle David, an Episcopal minister, is wearing his black clothes and white collar. He's the second oldest brother. David's daughter Kathy is his only child.

Uncle Peter, who is a doctor like my dad, is standing next to him. He is the third in line. Pete has four daughters: Barbie, Beth, Susan and Amy.

But Beau is here with me. It seems like his three older brothers are angry with him. I guess they need someone to blame. I'm starting to figure it out. Brain Doctor Beau couldn't fix what was going on with Berc's head. So, he recommended an institution instead of a treatment. Woodson, David and Peter were disappointed in their little brother. His choice of profession was useless. I bet Beau is vowing, now, to prove them wrong. The way I do whenever he calls me "buzzard tail."

Beau has been teaching me about baseball and teams. I think Beau's brothers just kicked him off the Bercaw team. Grandmother probably should be the umpire but she can't judge her own children. She's being pulled from side to side. I curl up next to my dad. He puts his arm around me. We're a team: he and I.

I look around at all my cousins. They look frozen. My cousin Nancy sees me, and smiles. I wish we could go swimming in the river at the farm after this is over, but it's cold and blustery. I look down at the ugly wool coat that one of the cousins brought for me to wear on this occasion. We don't need coats in Florida where Mom, Dad and I live now, again, after our foray into Alabama.

Beau is part of a private practice in Largo. He has a big fancy office, and wears a white lab coat that says "Dr. Bercaw, Neurology" in black script. When my mother calls him, she tells the secretary that she is "Mrs. Dr. Bercaw." I must be Miss Dr. Bercaw.

The pastor is reading from the Bible. I can tell it's my grandmother's

Bible because I see the gold lettering on the front that says Nannie Dunlap, which was my great-grandmother's name, and Nancy S. Bercaw—the S for Scott—who is my grandmother.

I wish I had been named Beth, Susan, Kathy, Amy or Barbie like the other girl cousins. I am Little Nan. My cousin is Nancy. Grandmother is Grandmother. Great-grandmother was Nannie—although she died a long time ago. When someone yells "Nancy" at family gatherings, I never think of myself as the one they want.

My grandfather's full name was Woodson Woods Bercaw. He and Grandmother Nancy named their first-born son Woodson Woods Bercaw, too. But my uncle broke the pattern when he named his first-born son Woodson Scott Bercaw. Grandfather was furious because Virginia and Bercaw tradition had been compromised.

In my grandparent's Virginia, the first-born son was given his father's full name, as well as his entire inheritance, including the family farm. The rest of the children had to fend for themselves.

The service ends. We walk past Berc's grave on our way to the meeting room in the basement of Lyles Baptist Church. Nearly everyone in Fluvanna County has come to pay their final respects to Berc and to see Grandmother and the brothers. I hear someone tell my father that putting Berc in a home was the right thing to do.

"He shoulda gone there a long time ago, Beau. Glad you finally talked sense into your mother."

My father nods. I notice another tear trying to escape. He swipes it away. I reach for his hand. I think he feels like he's done something wrong. I have that feeling all the time. Maybe it's another Bercaw legacy.

Beau bends down to look at me.

"You're a good ol' gal," he says. "Just like your grandmother."

My cousin Nancy comes over and asks if I would like to go play outside for a while. Beau says it's a great idea. I let go of his hand and take my cousin's. As soon as we leave the building, we start running. All the cousins are playing hide and seek among the gravestones and trees. Our fancy clothes are getting dirty, but we're pretty sure no one will care.

"We could run around naked and the grown-ups wouldn't pay us no mind," cousin Kathy says. Her dad is Uncle David, the Episcopal minister. He was thrown out of Virginia Military Institute after a hazing event more extreme than the school had ever seen.

David had been the *victim* of this brutality, not the perpetrator. Supposedly, it was payback for the considerable sins of his big brother Woodson, who graduated from VMI a few years earlier and become a Lieutenant Colonel in the Army, Tank Commander, Armor Division.

David transferred to Bluefield College in West Virginia and emerged as a minister. No one ever told me the details. No one ever told me anything. That's what it means to be a Bercaw. You have to figure everything out for yourself. And when you have the answers, you don't share them.

We all take a break from the game to look at Berc's grave.

WOODSON

WOODS

BERCAW

Virginia
Captain
3 Cavalry
World War I & II
Korea

May 22, 1896
January 7, 1971

"What is the cavalry?" I ask. "Did he ride around on horses?" Everyone shrugs.

"Why isn't there a quote or a poem or something?" asks cousin Beth.

"Bercaws don't like words," answers cousin Nancy. "Just numbers, war and the occupied countries of the Pacific Ocean."

Cousin Susan accidentally drops her Coke can on top of Berc's grave. A little bit of the brown soda spills out on the fresh brown topsoil.

"You've cursed us," says Nancy. And we all run as fast as we can back to Lyles, some of the younger cousins scream bloody murder. We rush inside to find our parents.

Beau and my mom are sitting with the Lovings, Grandmother's best friends in the county.

"Do you think your mother will stay on the farm?" Harriet Loving is asking my dad.

"I hope so," Beau answers meekly. "I sure do love the farm."

"Dad," I interrupt. "Excuse me, but I need to talk to you."

"What is it, Gal?"

"It's private."

Beau and I walk over to the pie table. He gets another piece.

"Dad, one of the cousins spilled Coke on Berc's grave. Are we cursed now? Forever?"

My dad smiles real big for the first time in weeks.

"Gal, Bercaws have been cursed long before today."

CHAPTER THREE

HARBOR VIEW LANE
LARGO, FLORIDA

My father is reading *The Little Mermaid* to me. It is the fall of 1972. I am nearly seven.

"There dwell the Sea King and his subjects."

I am sitting on his lap on a bamboo couch on the lanai of our Florida home. I have learned our address: 310 Harbor View Lane. We live in a fishbowl—long sliding glass doors in every room facing the water. People who walk through our backyard or front yard can see us. At night, I use a flashlight to get to the bathroom instead of turning the lights on because I'm scared of who's out there. Of course, I'm scared of who's in here too.

The sun hasn't set yet, and I look out at the inlet that runs through our neighborhood and into the Gulf of Mexico. The house is quiet. My mother is finishing the dishes. She never, ever leaves one plate dirty overnight. She is pregnant. The baby is due soon. I'm hoping for a sister.

My father keeps reading.

> They were six beautiful children; but the youngest was the prettiest of them all; her skin was as clear and delicate as a rose-leaf, and her eyes as blue as the deepest sea; but, like all the others, she had no feet, and her body ended in a fish's tail.

I pull my legs together tightly, turn my feet out and pretend I have a long beautiful turquoise tail fin. I live with my father, the Sea

King, under the water, safe from all the horrible things on land—
like Berc's illness and family curses.

Daddy keeps reading.

> Your tail will then disappear, and shrink up into what mankind
> calls legs, and you will feel great pain, as if a sword were passing
> through you.

"Daddy, is that true?" I ask. "Is that really in the book or are you
making that part up? Don't tell me she's facing a curse like Bercaw!"

"Gal, she has to give up her tail to love the prince and be human.
There is a price for any kind of love."

"Why would anyone want to become human?" I say. "Life on land
is scary, right, Daddy?"

"Yes, but we must learn to be brave. That is the meaning of life—
be ye mermaid or human."

"Keep reading, Daddy. None of this makes any sense to me."

"It will, Gal. It will. I promise."

Beau goes back to the book. The Little Mermaid loves the prince
but she can't actually tell him because she gave up her voice, as well
as her fin, for a chance to marry him.

"Dad! That's not right. What does he have to give up?"

My father laughs. "Let me keep reading and we'll find out."

"Wait a minute! What if I promise never to marry a prince, or anyone—can I get my legs turned into a fin? You know, the opposite
of what she did?"

"Unfortunately, it doesn't work that way," Beau says. "But I like
that idea, Gal."

Night has fallen; my mother has gone to sleep. I can no longer
see the water in the distance. Beau kisses me on the top of my head,
and keeps reading until the very end of the book.

> The little mermaid drew back the crimson curtain of the tent,
> and beheld the fair bride with her head resting on the prince's

breast. She bent down and kissed his fair brow, then looked at the sky on which the rosy dawn grew brighter and brighter; then she glanced at the sharp knife, and again fixed her eyes on the prince, who whispered the name of his bride in his dreams. She was in his thoughts, and the knife trembled in the hand of the little mermaid: then she flung it far away from her into the waves; the water turned red where it fell, and the drops that spurted up looked like blood.

I sob into my father's chest. "I've never heard anything so horrible. She should have put the dagger in the prince's chest and gotten her tail back. Instead, the Little Mermaid disappears into nothing. She drowns. I can't stand it. Why are you reading this to me?"

"She let him live because she loved him."

"She died because she loved him, Dad. It's different."

"I guess you are right, Gal."

My father tucks me into bed and sits down next to me.

"Let's say a prayer," he says.

"Yes, let's pray to God that we don't drown, and that I don't fall in love with a selfish prince. Right, Dad?"

"Right, Gal."

Beau begins.

"Dear God, we pray tonight for all the people lost at sea. And for all the people whose brains are lost in their own cerebral fluid. Help us live and love while we can. To make sacrifices for other people. To save people from suffering as best we can. Please help me raise young Nancy to be a person as good as her grandmother. Give her the strength that she needs to grow up in the world, and to help me one day when I need her to make decisions about my life. Amen."

My father has been even stranger since Grandpa Berc's death. He is talking less and less to my mother and me. He works really hard at the office and hospital, and comes home very late. We go visit sometimes and bring him a tuna sandwich. Dad is very particular about what he eats. No eggs. No fat. No white bread. He makes me take vitamins every day. None of my friends have even heard of vitamins, which is okay because I've never heard of this Fonz they are always discussing.

The last time Mom and I were at his office, I noticed that he had a brain in a jar in the middle of his huge desk—a desk handcrafted to his specifications in Baguio, the Philippines. I had picked up the jar and examined the contents. It looked smaller than I imagined brains would. It seemed to be missing a slice or two, like a piece of roast beef.

"PUT THAT DOWN!" my father yelled as he came in the room. I fumbled with the jar, and nearly dropped it.

"You ol' buzzard tail, Gal!" He grabbed the jar from me. "You damn well better pray this isn't damaged."

I backed away from my father, and out of his office, as he inspected the jarred brain.

My mother was talking with the nurses in the main office. I grabbed her arm and pulled her to the door. "We have to go, Mom. Now!"

"I want to finish reading this letter from your father to Grandmother, it's about Grandfather's illness."

She showed me the letter. The secretary had just finished transcribing it.

I want to write you regarding your inquiry about Berc's death. I don't know whether you will get a death certificate or not. I did get a copy of the autopsy report. The cause of death was pneumonia. The actual mechanism of death, no doubt was a cardiac irregularity. When I was in Roanoke, I was quite impressed with the staff up there and there was no doubt in my mind that he received excellent care. I think you should have no reservations about having him put in the VA Hospital. Regarding the brain, it may be some months before we have a final answer... As soon as we have it evaluated, I will be informed and will review the pathology myself.

My dad didn't come out of his office to say goodbye or to tell me if the brain was okay. He just went on to his next patient. Mom and I went home, stopping for milkshakes at McDonald's because Beau wouldn't be home for dinner.

"Why is Dad the way he is?" I asked her.

"He's just worried, Nan. He's got a lot of people with sick brains to fix."

"Does he love us?"

"Yes, of course. He's busy. A doctor belongs to a lot of people, not only his family. Our job is to share his gift of helping people. It's work for us too."

I want to tell my mother that we're more like his patients. We need more of him to get better.

A week later, Beau is sitting on the edge of my bed and praying for me to take care of him when the time comes. I want to ask who is going to take care of me if something happens to him, but I don't. Our lives are all mixed up with death. Pretty much like *The Little Mermaid*. A story that sounds sweet and lovely but turns out to be scary and ugly.

"Sometimes, Daddy, I have no idea what you're talking about. You should write fairy tales if doctoring doesn't work out."

"Your ol' dad sure loves you." He kisses me on the top of my head.

"Dad, I have a question."

"I hope I have the answer." He smiles really big at me.

I smile back. "What happened to Berc's brain?"

"Make an appointment to come see me and we'll discuss it."

Beau leaves the room. He shuts the door gently. I'm so mad that I try to wipe his kiss off my head with the pillow, and then I scream into it: *We don't talk about anything in this house.*

Wait, I tell myself. *Maybe not talking about Berc's brain keeps us safe from whatever happened to it.*

A few days later, Beau decides to join a private club—the kind he had sworn in Huntsville, Alabama, that he would never join. He heard that the best swim coach on the west coast of Florida works at Carlouel Yacht Club, which gives Beau a reason to cross the class line. Dick Smith was churning out champions in waves, especially sprinters, of which I was one. The Sea King is willing to do anything to keep his little mermaid in the water. After his finances are reviewed, and after he writes a big check, we are members. My mother is ecstatic.

I get faster and faster in the pool. Beau keeps track of all my times in his head. He knows when I drop even a fraction of a second. "Gal, you swam 14.5 at the dual meet in Sarasota. You just swam two-tenths under that. You are only four-tenths off the state record. If you keep improving at this rate, you'll break the record in two months."

My mother does all the shuttling to and from swim practices and to meets around the state despite the fact that she has a full-time job as a teacher. She loves Carlouel, though, and its prestigious members: the DuPont family; the Eckerds of Eckerd Drugs; and Dean Young, who is the artist of the *Blondie* comic strip. My mother is with her kind of people again. Mom helps organize swim meets and works as a race timer. She cheers me on with a big smile on her face and she wears cute swimsuits with built-in skirts. Other men notice her pretty tan legs. I wish I had her coloring instead of Beau's pinkness.

But there is a terrible side effect of joining Carlouel Yacht Club— my father becomes more stubborn about money. When paper towels go on sale at the drug store, with a limit of three rolls per person, Beau makes the three of us go in separately to buy our allotment. He demands to see receipts for everything my mother purchases. He chastises her for not finding the cheapest place to buy milk. I assume that we have been plunged into poverty because I swim so fast.

It's my fault. That's what Beau had said about his father's troubles. Maybe Bercaw children are the source of the curse. We bring it to the surface.

"Pride must suffer pain," I remembered the old grandmother mermaid telling the Little Mermaid, when she complained about the giant oyster shells attached to her tail fin as adornment.

26

My father is punishing us for the privilege of joining the club. Every step on dry land requires some suffering in return. The faster I get, the more we have to give up. No new clothes. No chocolate sauce for our ice cream. When we travel to swim meets, Beau says we can't afford hotels and have to camp instead.

My coach protests when the stakes are high.

"Dr. Bercaw, Nancy should sleep in a bed before competing in the Junior Olympics. She has a chance to win at least five events."

"The ground toughens her up," Beau answers, putting his arm around me. "She'd win no matter what she slept on."

I grin at my coach. It's not the ground that toughens me up. It's my dad, and I sense that he is training me for something greater than the 50-yard freestyle. Trophies are just one way into Beau's heart and out of my lonely sea. The other ways I haven't learned yet.

CHAPTER FOUR

THE TREE HOUSE

LARGO, FLORIDA

"Gal, I'm going to build you a tree house."

"Where?"

"In the backyard."

I am nine, and it is 1975. I am excited by the idea of my own hide-out, away from my three-year-old brother, Lee, who likes to chase me with the plastic chainsaw Beau gave him.

The tree house will give me a place to hide from Lee—and, come to think of it, my father. Is that why Beau is building it?

I start organizing the things I will take inside: sleeping bags, a brown box that I will pretend is a television, the *Merck Manual* so I can keep up my private medical studies, as well as pillows and some blankets.

I also have some *Tiger Beat* magazines that a friend has given me, although I don't recognize any of the teenage stars in the pictures. I can identify William F. Buckley, Jr., and Jacques Cousteau, but pop stars like the Partridge family are not on my radar. The only reason I know anything about them is because, on several occasions, my friends at St. Paul's Episcopal School tell me that my haircut resembles David Cassidy's.

Most people, though, say that I look exactly like my father. *How can a nine-year-old girl look like her thirty-seven-year-old father?* Things are making less sense to me as I get older. I can't help but wonder if I am getting Grandfather's disease.

Beau has hired one of his patients, who can't pay his medical bills, to build the tree house. I watch the carpenter carefully because school is out for summer. I swim early in the morning and late in the afternoon, but I have the middle part of the day to play and worry.

The carpenter makes the stilts and the cross beams, then the four walls, then the corner posts and then the roof. There doesn't seem to be anything wrong with the carpenter. So I wonder why he went to see my dad in the first place. But I look closer at his hands when he is sawing. They shake a little bit.

I ask my mother why the carpenter is shivering. It's more than 95 degrees outside.

"Parkinson's disease," she says.

"Are we allowed to say that in front of Dad?"

"Yes, that one is okay."

Every day, I ask the carpenter how much longer it will take to complete my tree house.

"Not sure," he says. "The directions are fairly complex."

"He's real good," my father comments during his evening inspection of the progress. "Doesn't matter how long it takes, as long as it's safe."

"When he's done, can I have one of his sawhorses so I can pretend it's a real horse?" I ask Beau.

"Don't be greedy, Gal. Be grateful for the tree house."

I nod, ashamed of myself.

After two weeks of waiting and watching, the tree house is declared complete. The carpenter leaves me both sawhorses, saying that the area underneath the tree house makes a fine stable for them.

When he leaves, I realize there's no ladder for me to get inside. From the ground, all I can do is look up at a square trapdoor hole in the floor.

I ask my mother for a ladder, but she says that I have to wait until Beau gets home for the grand opening.

"Can I sleep up there tonight?" I ask her.

"Let's see what your father says." She goes back to polishing the silver.

When I hear Beau's car pull in the driveway, I run out to greet him.

"It's done! The tree house is done! But there is no ladder! I really want to go in! Can I stand on your shoulders? Come on, come see."

"Hold on, Gal," he says. "I have to get something out of the trunk first."

I go to the back of the car to help him, thinking that he has probably stocked up on paper towels or toilet paper if he's seen them on sale somewhere.

Beau opens the trunk and pulls out a rope ladder.

"Is that for me?"

"Yes, I wanted you to have a rope ladder so you could pull it up and no one else could have entry unless you said so."

"Can we put it in now?"

"Yes," he says.

We walk around the side of our house to my tree house, which has been erected amongst a group of palm trees not too far—but far enough—from the back door.

My mom brings the painter's ladder from the garage, and my father puts it under the hole. My brother runs around the backyard screaming, "Me! Me! Me!"

Beau goes up first. He secures the rope ladder on the hooks that the carpenter has installed.

"Gal, you can come up now," he says.

I look at my mother, who is smiling. My brother finally calms down and stands next to her blowing bubbles. It's like they've come to see me set sail for the Philippines.

I pull myself up the ladder until my head passes through the opening. Beau is sitting on the floor of the tree house grinning ear to ear. He reaches out his hand and pulls me the rest of the way inside. I sit next to him wondering if he'll ever explain this thing to me.

"I had one as a kid," he says a minute later.

"On the farm?"

"Yup. Not as nice as this. Just some boards in a tree."

"Mom told me that the builder had Parkinson's disease."

"That's right, Gal. He did."

"Is he gonna get better?"

"The sad truth is no. Very few of my patients get better. I just try to postpone the end and then make it easier for them."

"Is Parkinson's the worst thing a person can get?"

"No, Gal. What your grandfather had was worse, in my opinion, although I suspect some folks would disagree with me. Parkinson's is a neuro-degenerative disease, too. Alzheimer's starts with memory loss. Parkinson's begins with gait issues. They both eat away at your brain. And any sickness that takes your life before you're dead is too horrible to imagine. It's not a contest."

"Dad, isn't there some medicine? Like Penicillin?"

"No, in these cases, something else is at work. Not a bug. Brains turn against themselves. Rot or clog from the inside. We just don't know how or why."

We stand up—my father hunches over in the close confines—and look across our neighbors' yards, down to the Gulf of Mexico.

"Can I sleep up here tonight?" I ask.

"I guess so," he says. "When you go to bed, though, pull the ladder up and close the trap door. There's a little hook you can use to lock it."

I realize instantly that my father had instructed the carpenter-patient how to do everything, from the latch and the hook to the open windows with a view in every direction. He even told him to leave the sawhorses for me.

Mom announces that it's time for dinner. Beau and I ease down the rope ladder. We step back a few yards and take a good look at the final product.

I put my hands on my hips and stare at the structure. What is this thing? It's not a tree house. Maybe it's a fort—a replica of a military fort at some far-flung outpost, like the ones I've had a glimpse of on *M*A*S*H*. I used to walk into the living room when my father was watching the TV show and claim that I needed a glass of water, just to see what was making him laugh so hard.

Then it hits me. I have seen buildings like this before. Every summer on the way to Virginia, we stop at as many Civil War battlefields as possible. Fort Sumter. Harper's Ferry. Appomattox. Chancellorsville. New Market. Gettysburg. Fredericksburg. Spotsylvania. Shiloh.

The First and Second Campaigns in Manassas are Beau's favorite battles because of the Confederate army's sizable victories, led first by General P.G.T. Beauregard and General Stonewall Jackson (who earned his nickname there), and then again by Jackson and General Robert E. Lee.

I look at the tree house again.

Oh my God.

I realize what my father has done.

U.S. Air Force Captain Beauregard Lee Bercaw—son of Cavalry Captain Woodson Woods Bercaw—has built a miniature Civil War signal tower in our backyard.

I put my head in my hands. For one second, I believed that he was acting like a normal dad and we were a normal family.

Maybe even like Shelly Kapalack's family, who owned the Travelodge Hotel in Clearwater near the Scientology headquarters. Shelly went to St. Paul's School with me. The Kapalacks lived in three rooms on the first floor of the hotel. They had plain old bureaus, chairs and desks, and hung pictures like "Christina's World."

Their house was the polar opposite of ours, which is decorated with Oriental carpets, hand-carved wood tables, bamboo chairs, temple rubbings, and pictures of the Taj Mahal. I never want to invite anyone over because our Asian artifacts embarrass me. I don't know how to explain our taste. I greatly preferred the simplicity of life and furniture at the Travelodge.

Whenever I visited Shelly, we got to ride the elevator and work behind the front desk with her dad. He greeted guests with a big smile and hugged Shelly after she handed the key over the counter.

That's what I wanted: regular affection and living quarters, not a dad who was obsessed with old wars, glass houses and brain diseases.

After dinner, Beau hoists my sleeping bag and flashlight up to me, along with a Snickers bar and a copy of *Swiss Family Robinson*.

"Don't stay up too late, and don't wear the battery down. Always have power left in case of emergencies."

"Don't worry, Dad, I'll be fine."

"Wait, I got you something else, too."

I stick my head out of the hatch and look down at him. "What?"

"Walkie-talkies," he says, and passes one up to my dangling hand. "Call me if you need anything."

"Thanks, Dad, this is amazing." I close the hatch.

"Your ol' dad sure loves you," I hear him mumble from the other side.

I open the hatch up a crack and say, "I love you too."

A few days later, my father gets a letter in the mail from the neighborhood association. They inform him that tree houses are against the bylaws and covenants, and that he has fourteen days to remove it from our premises or else he will be fined.

Beau reads me the letter and then rips it up. My mom looks nervous.

A month later, he receives another letter saying that he owes $100 in fines and that the structure must be removed or the association will have it removed. Beau sends them a letter in response.

Dear Sirs,

I will not remove the tree house, nor will I pay this fine. This is my property and I shall do as I please on it. I have a covenant with God, who protects my freedom, and it trumps your covenant to protect the neighborhood from evil tree houses.

Sincerely,
General George Washington

My mother pleads with him to take the tree house down and to respect the neighborhood rules, which enrages Beau.

"I will not surrender my rights for these people who have nothing better to do than snoop around and see who's breaking their idiotic rules. If they tear it down, I will build a bigger one in the front yard."

A few nights later, the phone rings. It's the president of the association. I listen as Beau speaks to him.

"Jim, I will not take the tree house down. It is for my daughter. I won't remove it because a few people think it's an eyesore. It has a purpose and it's on my property."

Jim speaks for a short while before Beau chimes in more angrily.

"Here's the deal. I will paint it green so it blends in better. That's my only concession. If anyone comes to try and take it away, like thieves, I will have no other choice than to protect my land and my family with the weapons I keep for this purpose."

It's Jim's turn. I have no idea what he is saying, but my father is giving me the thumbs up.

"Good," Beau says. "I'll paint it on Sunday instead of taking out the boat. If anyone from the association wants to come by and help, we'd be grateful."

Beau hangs up the phone and laughs like a hyena.

"We did it, Gal. We won. Freedom reigns. Yee-haw!"

The next day, he gets an old cowbell from the garage and hangs it from the ceiling in the fort.

"Ring it real loud," Beau says. "Proclaim liberty throughout the land."

He keeps his promise to Jim, and we spend all day Sunday painting the outside of the tree house an Army green. We stop only to sip from the canteens of water Beau has purchased to keep us from getting parched.

"What was your dad like?" I ask when we finish. "Before he got sick."

"He loved his country, Gal. Let's go to my den, I want to show you something."

We walk into his private office in the back of the house, behind Lee's bedroom. I'm not usually allowed in there, but sometimes I snoop around. There are lots of medical textbooks and journals piled high. There's a pink corduroy couch where Beau likes to sit and read. He also has a spinal column dangling from an IV hook positioned next to the couch so he can think about various vertebrae injuries.

When a boy we knew from Carlouel was injured in a waterskiing accident, Beau used the spinal column to show me why the kid would be in a wheelchair for the rest of his life.

"Injury in C1-C4 level, Gal. He'll need help for everything."

Today, Beau has something else in mind. He pulls a small dinner plate with gold trim out of the back of a filing cabinet. He hands it to me. There's a Confederate flag on the front with the phrase "Land We Love" underneath.

"Turn it over," Beau says.

The other side reads:

> Produced by
> Woodson W. Bercaw
> Manager
> Stage Junction
> Virginia, US

I hand the delicate plate back to my dad—not entirely sure what the image means or what secret we are keeping. Why does Beau want to hide proof of grandfather's plate business in the back of a filing cabinet? I'm beginning to think that people lose their minds because they can't comprehend their parents—not the other way around.

CHAPTER FIVE

INTRACOASTAL WATERWAY
GULF OF MEXICO, FLORIDA

"Let's go for a boat ride," Beau says to my brother and me. It's a Sunday afternoon, the one day a week he isn't on call. It is 1976, and the fire hydrants in town are painted red, white and blue in honor of the Bicentennial.

I am eleven and my biceps are bulging from my swim training. I look more like a boy than my five-year-old brother does. I'm not happy about it, but at least I am swimming faster than ever. I'm not sure how I'll ever be a lady anyway because my dad seems hell-bent on making a man out of me. Those are his exact words.

My mom stopped going on these boat outings a few months ago after the Great Shoe Incident—in which my brother accidentally dropped one of Beau's topsiders into "the drink," as Dad called the water between the boat and the dock.

"Never, ever pass things over the drink," he had warned on numerous occasions. "Make sure the exchange takes place over the dock or the boat. Not over the water."

Poor Lee had forgotten the rule and dropped the shoe mid-pass to me.

"Get it," Beau screamed, pushing Lee into the drink. Lee wasn't a very good swimmer anyway, but the murky water and muddy bottom hampered him even further. Lee, sobbing every time he surfaced, couldn't find the shoe, let alone breathe. I pulled him out of the water.

Beau ran up the hill and into our house. He grabbed one of Lee's

36

brand-new sneakers—the ones he got instead of an Easter basket—and ran back to the dock. Beau threw the sneaker as far as he could into the canal. Lee ran to his room and refused to come out for dinner. I pushed an Oreo under his door. He pushed it back out.

While we're out at sea, these days, Mom, dressed in a white Izod shirt and a tiny white skirt, plays tennis with the neighborhood ladies. Sometimes they play bridge instead and have tiny cucumber sandwiches with sips of dry sherry.

After each trip, Lee and I have to make sure the boat is perfectly clean for the next ride. Beau worries that barnacles could destroy the great Garuda—our 20-foot Bertram with an inboard/outboard motor and a small sleeping cabin. Beau named the boat Garuda because of his affection for Hindu gods.

Garuda, part bird and part deity, was Lord Vishnu's massive mount. Garuda was also the sworn enemy of Naga, the serpent race. Hindus believe that Vishnu is the Preserver of the World. Brahma is the Creator. Shiva is the Destroyer of Evil.

"It takes all three," Beau explains, "to keep life in balance. Sort of like God, Jesus and Satan. Just the way the United States has three government branches: the legislative, the judicial and the executive. That was the genius of the great Virginians, Jefferson and Madison. They took what they learned about the world and religion and applied it to the Constitution."

On this occasion, my father lets me bring along Beth, a friend from the neighborhood. He feels sorry for her. Beth's mother had called us one morning and said her husband had died in his sleep. Beau told her not to call the paramedics because it would cost a lot of money. He went over to confirm her findings and called a funeral home.

"No sense, Gal, in paying for a paramedic when someone is dead. It's robbery. Plus it creates more work in the ER. Dead people need to go directly to funeral homes."

Mom sends us off with peanut butter sandwiches in baggies and lemonade in a big Thermos. Beau rarely allows us to have sodas. He did authorize an annual root beer float at a certain diner off I-95 on our way to Virginia each summer, the cold sugary drink offered up as the lone antidote to our un-air-conditioned van.

Before every boating trip, Beau drives to the 7–11 to get additional "provisions," which is code for Snickers bars. Snickers bars are a very serious business in my father's mind. They have peanuts for protein to "hold us over" in case we get lost at sea for a few days.

But "dumb-dumbs" are his main concern—those wayward boaters who don't know, or choose not to follow, the rules of the United States Power Squadrons. By age ten I had already passed two courses in boating safety with the local chapter. My father, who framed the certificates for my wall, wanted me to be able to steer Garuda in case he should fall prey to a "cerebral infarction," like Beth's father had, while we were in the middle of a busy channel.

"You won't be able to save me, Gal, but you've got to get yourselves home."

His second worry was lightning.

"You are more likely to be killed by lightning than a shark," he said after we saw *Jaws*.

The day we go boating with Beth is clear and calm. Beau also brings our dog, Heidi, a miniature schnauzer, along for the ride. Heidi barks at anything, even a falling leaf. I think my dad wants to see how she will react to the Gulf of Mexico. Beau can squeeze a science experiment into any outing.

Beau motors slowly out of the canal in our neighborhood, which is well marked with "no wake" signs. The cement seawalls that keep the water off our lawns are cracked and fragile. Repairing them is very expensive.

Once we're in the Intracoastal Waterway, Beau picks up speed. Beth and I are allowed to ride in the front of the boat, as long as our legs are tucked in the hatch that drops a few feet into the cabin. Under no circumstances can we dangle our limbs off the bow.

We like to look out ahead of Garuda. We take turns calling out the numbers on the markers, and looking for cute boys in passing boats. Beau tells us to holler if any dumb-dumbs encroach.

Lee rides shotgun to our father, who sits behind the boat's slightly corroded metal steering wheel. Lee is expected to hand our father provisions as necessary. Today, he is also trying to stop Heidi from barking at the seagulls overhead. Beth and I can hear them over Garuda's loud motor.

Lee is screaming, "No, Heidi, no."

"Both of you be quiet," Beau yells.

Beth goes to help Lee control Heidi. I resume my lookout.

Garuda is headed directly for one of the huge wooden channel markers. I'm not sure if I need to say anything to Beau or not. He is so vigilant about his boating. If I accuse him of not paying attention, he will yell at me too.

I look back at him. Beau is reading an ocean chart. He has slowed the boat down a bit. He knows what he's doing. There must be some shallow water nearby. It's low tide. If Garuda runs aground, there will be hell to pay.

The marker is getting closer. I calculate the distance based on the twenty-five-yard pool I train in every day. There is half a pool left until we'll hit it.

"Dad!" I scream, and look for him. Beau's head is turned away from the wheel. Lee is hitting Heidi on the head. Beth is trying to stop him.

I brace myself for a crash.

The sound is like an oak tree falling over into a lake: a loud creak, and then a huge splash.

The whole front fiberglass hull of Garuda curls forward and opens up. Some of the fiberglass hits me, like shrapnel.

Lee lets out a blood-curdling scream. Heidi has gone overboard, as have all our provisions. Lee seems more concerned about the Snickers bars than our dog. Beth looks fine, albeit shocked.

I jump in and get Heidi.

"Swim to the front, Gal, and assess the damage," Beau instructs me after I pass Heidi back into the boat. Another boat is making its way toward us. I worry about it running me over, and getting chopped up by the motors—which Beau told me happens from time to time. He had seen it in the ER, along with spinal fractures from the cervical to the sacral, as well as every kind of traumatic head injury. Even decapitation.

I am relieved that all the damage has been to the top of Garuda. She isn't going to sink. I swim back to the ladder and pull myself in.

The other boater pulls up and asks Beau if we're okay.

"We're fine," he says. "The impact felled the engine."

"Can we take you home?" the boater asks.

"No, I don't want to leave the boat," Beau says. "I'll radio the Coast Guard for a tow."

The other captain says, "Good luck," and motors off.

"Gal," Beau turns to me. "Eat a Snickers bar."

"I'm not hungry," I say. In fact, I feel sick to my stomach.

"You're going to need your strength."

I look up at him. There is a little bit of blood dripping down from his brow into his big blue eyes.

"Dad, what happened? Where are your glasses?" I use my forefinger to wipe the blood away.

"They smashed my face and flew out of the boat."

He can't see anything nearby without them.

"Gal, I need you do to something."

"Aren't we gonna call the Coast Guard?" I ask, worried that he has forgotten the plan. Did the impact injure Beau's brain? Did he just come down with Alzheimer's disease? Is that how it happens? Bang, you've got it. Suddenly the dumb-dumb you feared is yourself.

"I don't want to bother them," he says, as if we were all dead and the paramedics weren't necessary. "Besides, we're less than a mile from home."

"How are we gonna get there, Dad?"

"You're going to pull us, Gal."

"What?" I shiver.

Beth's and Lee's jaws drop open.

"Tie this line around your waist. Then, tie the other end of it to the notch at the low front part of the helm. The hook used for towing."

"Then what?"

"Start swimming." Beau hands me the line. "Use the kind of knots that the Power Squadrons taught you. I can't see to do it myself."

Beth starts to cry. Lee hands me a soggy Snickers that he pulled out of the water after the impact. I eat it.

I want to say *no* to my father, but I can't. He'll tell me I'm stupid. And the one thing you don't want to be, as a Bercaw, is stupid. Instead, you must silently overcome obstacles. I must endure Beau to earn his love.

"Dad, this is my brand-new Speedo," I argue, appealing to his frugality. He had bought the red-white-and-blue, stars-and-stripes swimsuit for my most recent appearance at the Junior Olympics.

"I'll buy you a new one," he snaps. "And if you do this, you don't have to go to swim practice for a week."

"But I like swim practice," I counter. "I don't want to miss it."

"Gal, stop it. You're pulling us. Ready. Set. Go."

I hop in the drink, defeated by Beau, yet comforted by the warm Gulf water. Beau puts up the flag that indicates we are a vessel under distress and being towed—by his eleven-year-old champion-swimmer daughter.

I pull Garuda out of the channel in less than fifteen minutes, swimming freestyle as fast as I can because I'm scared of being hit by someone who might not notice my scrawny tugboat self.

"Red, right, return," I chant to myself. The navigational mantra of the Power Squadrons: *The red channel markers will be on your right when returning from your trip.* I breathe in a little saltwater and choke. I am just like the Little Mermaid, sent back to the waves when her prince marries another. Maybe Beau is trying to teach me a lesson today. Maybe this wasn't an accident. Maybe this was his plan to test my readiness for what lies ahead.

I think about my last water adventure with him, only a few months before. We had gone to central Florida for a weekend of fun at Lake Okeechobee. We'd been swimming with lots of other families when the lifeguard suddenly blew his whistle and screamed, "Everybody out! There's a gator!"

I was close to shore and got on land quickly. I scanned the lake for Beau and Lee. They were smack dab in the middle of the lake with the gator headed toward them. The lifeguard was yelling, "Hurry, hurry!" Soon everyone else was out of the water, too, and holding their breath as they watched my father and brother race for their lives.

Beau was doing the backstroke with Lee on his chest.

"Kick, son, kick," my dad yelled, his arms wind-milling faster than I had ever seen. They had about twenty yards on the gator, but it was gaining on them. I could hear my brother crying.

The lifeguard rushed into the shallow water to help Beau and Lee out. The gator turned away. My father raised his hands into the air and loudly said, "We did it!" My brother fell in the sand sobbing. I put a towel over him and rubbed his back.

The lifeguard put up a red flag to indicate that the lake was closed. When my brother regained his composure, we walked back to our campsite.

"Watch out for quicksand," my father joked. "And sinkholes and spontaneous combustion."

Nothing you could see coming or control, just like Beau.

"Wish we could eat that gator for dinner," my dad said. I grabbed my brother's hand because he needed comfort and wasn't going to get it from Gator Man, as Beau was suddenly referring to himself.

Instead we had hotdogs and canned French-style green beans.

After one bite, Lee refused to eat the green beans. "They taste like slimy strings," he said, throwing his plastic fork into the sand.

"What?" my father snapped, eyes blazing. "I made that meal for you. Eat every bit of it."

"No."

"Yes."

"No.

"Yes."

"No."

"If you do not eat those beans, you will not get any Oreos."

"I don't care."

"You will not get any other food until you eat those beans."

"I'll never eat them," my brother said. He got up and went into the tent. Night had already fallen. With a flashlight, I looked for more sticks for the fire, and cleaned off Lee's fork.

My father carefully wrapped up Lee's beans and put them in the cooler. He opened the cookies and gave me two handfuls, plus a big glass of milk.

"We're eating the cookies now," Beau called out to my brother, who didn't answer. When I went to bed, I noticed that Lee had moved his sleeping bag to the other side of mine, as far from our father as possible.

The next morning, Beau put the cold beans out for Lee and started making grits. Lee sat down at the picnic table and stared at those beans until tears fell into the bowl. I looked over at my dad, who was whistling and whisking at the campfire.

"Lee," I whispered. "Eat those beans. There's no way out."

He started eating, and gagging.

"If you throw them up, it doesn't count," Beau said as he served me grits and an Oreo. My weeping brother tried to get the beans down as fast as possible, swallowing them whole so as not to taste them.

When Lee was done, my father gave him an Oreo. Nothing more was said, but Beau began calling Lee "Dr. No."

Now, here I am pulling Dr. Bercaw, Dr. No and half-orphan Beth, back to shore. I'm like P.T. Barnum bringing the freak show to town.

Safely inside my neighborhood's canal, I roll over to do the backstroke for a while. As my arms windmill more slowly, and my feet flutter gently, I study Garuda's damage. It's as if a cannonball had hit her.

I wonder what my live cargo has been doing while I swam us to safety.

As I near our dock, I stop for a while to tread water and await further instructions. I can't possibly pull the boat into its slip. The area around the dock is full of sharp barnacles and shells. My feet would be ripped to shreds. Ha! The Little Mermaid indeed: every step like walking on thousands of knives.

After hearing nothing from the back of the boat for a few minutes, I untie the line around my waist and swim back to the ladder. I pull myself out.

"Good job, Gal," Beau says with a yawn. He is sitting in a folding chair facing the stern. Lee is asleep on his lap. Beth is dozing in the cabin with Heidi. "You saved Garuda."

I saved you.

Thanks to my swimming, my father will escape a fate worse than death—having to tell the Coast Guard, and everyone else, that a lapse in his thinking caused this crash. We hit that marker for one reason and one reason only: Beau's mind had drifted.

CHAPTER SIX

GREAT WALL OF CHINA RESTAURANT
CLEARWATER, FLORIDA

"We're going for Chinese food tonight," Beau announces to my brother and me. It might be the strangest thing he has ever said. It is 1978. I am nearly thirteen and just beginning to understand that my father's complexities know no bounds.

We never go anywhere on a Sunday evening. Usually we watch the *Six Million Dollar Man* because Beau is fascinated by Steve Austin's bionic implants. Otherwise, Lee and I are allowed only three hours of television a week. Our choices must be from one of the following: *National Geographic, The Waltons, Little House on the Prairie, Fat Albert* or *Walt Disney's Movie of the Week*. Once our choices are circled in red in the *TV Guide*, they are written in stone. No changes are permitted—unless the Rev. Billy Graham has a special.

"The idiot box will rot your brain," my father claims. I picture melted gray matter pouring out of my ears like wax as John-Boy narrates life on Walton Mountain. Beau likes the Waltons because the real-life family is near the Bercaw farm in Palmyra. Some of the Waltons' kin attend Lyles Baptist Church, where Berc is buried, and where my grandmother still goes to services.

The only thing I know about China is that my father puts the word "Red" in front of it. I know a bit more about Japan because Grandfather wanted to re-join the Army to fight the country in World War II, even though he was getting a bit old for service and had a good high-paying job in Washington, D.C. He wrote to General Douglas MacArthur and asked to be called back into active duty.

45

April 9, 1941

Mr. Woodson W. Bercaw,
  1660 Hobart St., N. W.,
  Washington, D. C.

My dear Bercaw:

I have just received your Air Mail letter of
March 28th, expressing your patriotic desire to be re-
called to active service. Your application to that effect
should be made at once to The Adjutant General of the Army.
I suggest that this letter accompany the application as it
gives me an opportunity to unqualifiedly recommend you for
active assignment. Your long and highly creditable service
with the Treasury Department in which you have displayed
great tact, energy, and zeal, as well as a special capacity
for obtaining information, would admirably fit you for
assignment either in the Intelligence or Judge Advocate
branches of the Army in addition to your own commission
as a Cavalry officer.

It is most highly creditable to you that your
application for active service is made in spite of the
fact that it will cause a marked reduction in your government salary. If there is any further assistance that I can
give you please call upon me.

Sincerely yours,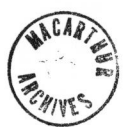

Berc was sent to learn Japanese in California, instead of being shipped out to the South Seas. Grandmother worked in a cannery there for a while before heading back to the farm with Beau, Peter and David. Young Woodson was busy making a name for himself at Virginia Military Institute.

In the parking lot of the Great Wall of China, which looks more like a temple than a wall, my brother asks a question.

"What do they have to eat?"

I sigh. *God, won't this kid ever learn? The number-one rule for being a Bercaw is: Don't challenge your dad.*

"We're not here for the food," Beau snaps. "Although I expect you to eat whatever is served. I want you to meet the owner of the restaurant. He's going to tell you about the horrors of Communist China and how grateful you should be for all you have."

"We are grateful," I say as sweetly as I can.

"Not enough," he says, unfolding himself out of the car.

Lee and I crawl out from the back seat. We each take one of our father's hands, unsure of what the man from China might do or say. I wondered if he would look like a Sasquatch. I certainly had more experience with a non-existent wild beast than with a real live person from China.

Beau was obsessed with Bigfoot, in the same way he was fixated on people from Communist countries. In the event that he actually found the hairy beast—and we did search for him whenever we were camping—we would probably be sitting down to hear about the horrors of being a solitary ape-man in North America. Suffering, in any form, interests my father to no end.

The Great Wall of China restaurant is dark inside. Strings of red lanterns hang from the ceiling. Each table has a candle inside a hollow Buddha. Murals of farmers and mountains and boats and temples decorate every wall. A man greets my father and takes us to a huge, round table with a place card that says, "Reserved for Bercaws."

Dad sits between Lee and me; four other chairs remain empty. Soon thereafter, another man comes over to the table and my father stands up.

"Dr. Bercaw, so glad you are here," the man says. "These must be your children."

"It's our honor to be here, sir," Beau says. "Nancy and Lee, please stand and greet Mr. Tan."

"We are very excited to be here, and to try your food," I manage to say. I am terrified that Dr. No will say something about beans.

"I will bring you the specialties of the house," Mr. Tan says.

"After we eat," Beau says, "would you kindly tell us about life in Communist China?"

Mr. Tan nods and bows. My father bows too. I curtsey like my mom has taught me. "Young women bow in China too," Mr. Tan says, smiling big. I bow.

I wonder how Beau met Mr. Tan, who seems healthy and fine. Surely he isn't a patient. I imagine Beau calling every Chinese restaurant in town and asking, "Did you escape from Communism?" and hanging up if the answer was no. Finally, perhaps, he happened upon Mr. Tan and now we are at his Great Wall restaurant. Maybe they met once, in a secret location, to strategize about how to turn ingrates into patriots.

"Two Shirley Temples," Beau says to a waiter. "And one Singapore Sling."

My drink arrives with a pink plastic mermaid hanging off the rim of the glass. My brother's cup has a green plastic bull straddling the rim. We smile for the first time this evening. Studying the placemats, Dad figures out which sign we are in the Chinese zodiac: Beau is a tiger; I am a snake; and Lee is a pig.

"A-ha!" Dad exclaims with each revelation.

"A-ha!" I repeat.

"Oink oink," adds Lee.

Two waiters deliver more food than I have ever seen in my life. Lee inhales fried chicken. Beau shovels rice and spicy broccoli into his mouth. I eat fried bean curd as if it were French fries.

"Can we come here all the time?" I ask Beau.

He nods, approvingly.

Mr. Tan sits down in one of the empty chairs. Beau wipes his mouth, and leans forward to listen.

"In China, I could not own a restaurant like this. I could not have this much food. There were rations. I could not pray to God. We had to be atheists. I was not free."

Beau watches him intently. His eyebrows rise and fall on Mr. Tan's words. When Mr. Tan says, "not free," my Dad's eyes water up. Mine follow suit because of Beau's sudden show of emotion, not from what Mr. Tan has said.

Mr. Tan continues for a long time. I hear the words he is saying, but they are heavily accented. *Mowh. Torchure.* I'm not sure what he means by them but I can tell it's bad, very bad.

My father understands everything. He is taking notes on a prescription pad, undoubtedly to quiz me later. He's done this before at Civil War battle sites and museums. He wants to see if I am paying attention. Whenever I don't remember what we've just learned, he says, "Gal, you've got to get this information through your thick skull."

Lee puts his head on the table and falls asleep. Beau doesn't seem to mind. I am so cold in Mr. Tan's air-conditioned restaurant that I put the red polyester napkins over my shoulders, which are sunburned from yesterday's swim meet. I now have all the girls' pool records at Carlouel.

"You are an amazing man," my father announces when Mr. Tan concludes an hour later. I wonder if there had been a dearth of amazing men in my father's youth, so he is hunting for proof that they actually exist—like Bigfoot.

At the farm one summer, Grandmother showed me a letter that Beau, who was five at the time, had written to Santa:

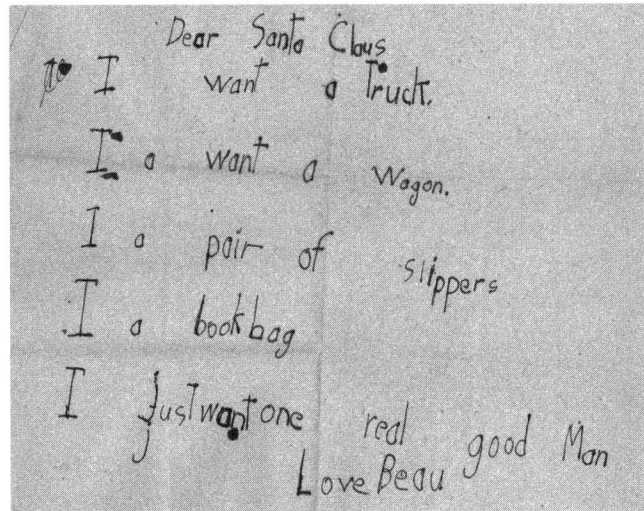

Grandmother didn't try to explain Beau's wish list to me; she just wanted me to see what my dad was like as a boy. I noticed that he tried to make a pattern for his wish list, yet by doing so he put an "a" in places where none was needed, and left out the word "want" in several spots. I made similar mistakes when learning to write.

But of greatest significance was what that little boy wanted: a good "Man" (with a capitalized "M")—as in good father? I wondered if my dad was trying to be that good man for me now. A good man who uses words frugally or perhaps has forgotten which to use where and when.

Upon finishing dinner at the Great Wall of China, we are given fortune cookies. Mine reads, "You will be blessed with great *luch*." I figure the typo means that I will always have bad luck. I must be bound for the People's Republic of China for being an ingrate; and my brother, the sleepy bean-hater, will be tortured by the scary *Mowh*.

I need to make things right before it's too late.

"Thank you for telling us this information and for feeding us this great food. When my brother loves a meal, he falls asleep. Kind of a disorder, please forgive him. But he is grateful too, just in his own way."

Beau pats me on the back, and looks sweetly at sleeping Lee.

Mr. Tan says, *"Zai jain."*

Dad carries my brother to the car. He lays Lee in the back, puts his suit coat over him, and stretches the seatbelt around him. I sit in the passenger's seat, which normally isn't permitted.

"A good man," my dad says on the way home. "God, the things people have to endure in this life. He's a very, very good man. You can learn a lot from a man like that, Gal."

CHAPTER SEVEN

CARLOUEL YACHT CLUB
CLEARWATER, FLORIDA

It is 1979 and I am fourteen. I want a summer job like a normal high school kid. Instead, I spend four hours a day in the pool at Carlouel. Mom drops Lee and me off in the morning and picks us up in the late afternoon. In between workouts, we drink milkshakes in the restaurant, play tennis and swim in the ocean with all the other kids who are dropped off as well. But I want to work at McDonald's. I want cash to see movies and to buy Gloria Vanderbilt jeans with gold piping down the side. I want to go on dates instead of trips to big swim meets in Ohio.

I summon all my nerve to ask Beau, over dinner, if I can get a part-time job. We rarely see him anymore. He is always at work. When he comes home, we don't know how to act. Lee wants to hide, but I tell him that's the cowardly way out. We have to face Beau, and act like everything is okay. We must be like Beau for him to love us.

My mother has dyed her hair blonde, and she has hired a housekeeper to help keep things in perfect order. The housekeeper's name is Angelo and he played soccer with Pelé in Brazil, before coming to America. Unfortunately, Angelo got injured and had to go to work cleaning houses. Beau approved because Angelo was down on his luck.

"How was practice today, Gal?" Beau asks when we sit down for dinner. He has just come home from the hospital. He hasn't even taken his lab coat off because he's going right back.

"Good. How was your day, Dad?" I ask, praying he is in the right frame of mind for my question. I had warned my mom of my plan.

"Bad. We have a patient with locked-in disease. I'll give anyone at this table $10 if they can tell me what that is."

"They're sick in a prison," Lee offers.

"Good guess, son," Beau says smiling. He respects wit, but despises sarcasm.

"Is the patient going to be okay?" I ask, painfully aware that the answer will determine whether I can bring up my interest in a job.

"Not unless I can come up with a cure before a stroke kills her."

"What is it, Dad? What's wrong with her?" Lee asks.

"'Locked in' means you are aware and awake but every part of your body is paralyzed except your eye muscles. You can think but can't communicate. People with it are terrified. I would say it's like being in hell while you're still alive. Or, worse yet, being buried in a coffin while you're still alive."

"Is it worse than what Berc had?" I ask, without thinking. My father stares at me with blazing eyes.

"How do you get it?" Lee asks, clearly frightened. I notice that he has moved all his vegetables to the outer rim of his plate. I wonder if Beau will notice.

"That's the second worst part," Dad says. "No one knows."

"What's the worst part?" I ask.

"No one has ever survived it."

"Beau, please don't scare Nancy and Lee," my mother interrupts, bravely. "Can we talk about something else? I think Nancy has something she wants to ask you."

"Go ahead, Gal. What do you want?"

I feel like I am locked in. I force myself to blink. I look at my hand holding the fork. I lift it to my mouth and take a bite of the grouper. Phew, I am okay.

"Dad, I would like to get a job."

"Your job is swimming. We pay a lot of money to belong to that club. You're worth it. One day, you'll get a scholarship to go to college. You are earning a living."

"I know, but couldn't I do something part-time?"

"Like what?"

"Well, maybe at McDonald's."

"You are not going to work at McDonald's. That's ridiculous. A world-class athlete doesn't spend her summer packaging Happy Meals. Why do you want a job anyway?"

"I would like to have money."

"For what? I get you everything you need."

"Like movie tickets. So I can go with my friends."

My father stares at me in disbelief. My mother gets up to clear the table. My brother runs to his room. I have no idea what's coming, but it's not going to be good.

Just recently I had snuck into a movie theatre—lacking the requisite funds or parental guidance—to see *Apocalypse Now*. What the big screen showed of the Vietnam War fascinated me. I imagined my father fixing up the injured soldiers flown to Clark Air Base in the Philippines. I realized why he couldn't stick around while my mother was in labor with me. He had soldiers to save from hellish wounds. Beau had heard about *Apocalypse Now* and its "anti-war" themes. I heard him cursing the movie to colleagues at Carlouel.

Beau stands up and puts his finger in my face.

"I took you to see *Chariots of Fire*, Gal, two weeks ago. You hated it, remember? You couldn't believe that Eric Liddell wouldn't compete on Sunday, even in the Olympics."

How would I ever forget? Beau called me an "idiot" for questioning Eric's motives as we left the movie.

"God is more important than your ideas," he chastised me in front of other people who were in line to see the film. He had shoved his forefinger into my temple in an attempt to get through to me, through to my ideas. I wanted to fight back, to say that being good at your sport, or your work, honors God too. But I couldn't. I wasn't even sure if that was true. My own thoughts succumbed to Beau's considerable cerebral force.

But now I am ready to fight back better, smarter.

"Dad, I just want to have my own money like my friends do. To pay my own way when I go places with them. Or, maybe just to buy a new book."

"I'll buy you whatever book you want," he snaps.

I retreat to my room. I stare at the poster of Bruce Springsteen on my wall. I had only heard his music at friends' houses. I wasn't allowed to listen to rock music. We listened to John Denver on long car rides. Beau played "Thank God I'm a Country Boy" over and over again.

One of my pals wished Bruce Springsteen was her boyfriend. But I wished Bruce were my dad.

I wished my biology teacher were my dad.

I wished my swim coach were my dad.

I wished Ernest Hemingway were my dad.

Anyone but the silent man who had the job of raising me and who worried more about locked-in disease than his own daughter's suffering. I had an acute case of locked-out disease.

Beau knocks on my door. I consider locking him out of my room, in honor of the disease of the day. "*Du jour*" as my mother would say when referring to soup at a fancy restaurant. Where is my mother right now? Why can't she stop him?

"Come in."

"Can I see your summer reading list?" he asks, calmly.

I hand it to him. It's on my desk with a copy of *Heart of Darkness* that I had gotten from the library. I turn the book over, so he can't see the title.

"I have an idea, Gal. I will pay you one penny per page you read this summer. That can be your job."

"Really? Can I read anything on this list?"

"You can read anything on this list or any other. Any book you want. You just have to write a short report on an index card in order to get your earnings."

"What about the books I already read this summer?"

"I'll pay for those too."

I'm feeling brave. "What about this one?" I ask, holding up Joseph Conrad's novel.

"That's a great book, Gal. Shame what that director did to the story in his *Apocalypse Now* movie. William F. Buckley, Jr. has a good piece about it in this week's *National Review*. Hey, I'll pay you for reading that article too. You can get paid for learning about capitalism. This way you can make money by learning that freedom isn't free. How's that for a deal?"

"Thank you, Dad, thank you so much."

"You're a buzzard tail, sweet Gal, but your ol' dad sure loves you." He puts his right arm around me and pulls me tight into his right side. His left hand pounds vigorously on my back.

Within a matter of days, I've earned $20. My mother takes me to the public library between swim practices. Beau's patient with locked-in disease gets worse. I overhear Beau on the phone telling her family that it's time to turn off life support.

"Let her die in peace," he says. I can tell there's a lump in his throat. "Not hooked up to machines. It's the right thing to do. There's no hope."

I look up locked-in disease at the library the next day. The official term for it is *cerebromedullospinal disconnection*. I think about Colonel Kurtz's dying words in Coppola's film and in Conrad's book, "The horror. The horror."

I leave the library with *To Kill a Mockingbird*. Mom and Lee are waiting for me in the car. I show her my latest selection.

Mom's mouth twists up. Her brow furrows.

"What?" I ask.

"I'll pay you double not to read that book."

"Why?"

"You shouldn't read things like that."

My mother doesn't like uncomfortable subjects. I can tell this must be a big one by her reaction. She has told me to stay home from high school if I catch wind of a race riot in the making.

"Mom, it's the '80s!"

Images of desegregation were stuck in her head. In the late '50s, young Barbara went on a date with the son of Federal District Court Judge John Paul, who had ordered black students admitted to Warren County High School in Front Royal, and to a high school and elementary school in Charlottesville. Many white people in Virginia had put up massive resistance to mixed-race education.

I flip to the end of the book to see the page count. I calculate that Dad will pay me $2.86 to read it.

"So, you'll give me six bucks not to read this book?"

"Yes."

"What will we tell Dad? It's on my reading list."

"Nothing. Just skip over it."

I tell her that I'll think about it, and spend nearly the entire night reading the book.

I write up my review on an index card and slide it under my dad's wallet. The book makes me think that Beau is more like Atticus Finch than Colonel Kurtz.

> Great book! A man stands up for what he believes. He never falters in his pursuit of the truth, which isn't what everyone else in the town thinks is the truth. In a world where it's hard to know what to believe, Atticus Finch is a good man. The book is 286 pages long. Please provide me with $2.86.
>
> Love, Scout

Mom takes me to the library the next day, and I return the book. Beau has already put the money on my desk. He wrote, "*Pride cometh before a fall,*" on the back of the index card. Was he talking about himself or me? I ripped up the index card and put it in the trash compactor.

"I'm glad you didn't read it," my mother says when I get back in the car after returning the book, handing me six dollars. I hesitate before taking the money, but then I put the cash in the side pocket of my swim bag. I tell myself that my other job this summer is to make my mother happy because Beau has floated so far away from us. He is clinging to that brain in a jar on his desk as if it were a life-preserver.

II

The Middle

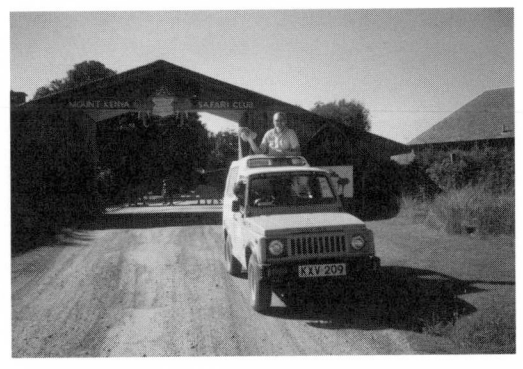

I am a brain, Watson.
The rest of me is a
mere appendix.

—Sherlock Holmes

(Sir Arthur Conan Doyle)

CHAPTER EIGHT

THE RIVANNA RIVER
PALMYRA, VIRGINIA

It is the summer of 1983. I am seventeen and have just finished my first year of college at the University of South Florida. I have a swimming scholarship, and I am studying English literature. Thanks to Beau and our penny-per-page deal, I have already read every book I've been asked to study.

We have come to Rebelanna for two weeks as we always do. But there is one big difference this year: my mother isn't with us; Beau's fiancée is.

"Canoe trip!" Beau hollers up the farmhouse stairs. My soon-to-be stepsister Kathy and I are just waking up in the room Beau had as a kid. My soon-to-be stepbrother Craig and my brother Lee are on the little porch in two small twin beds. We get dressed quickly in our swimsuits and T-shirts. I can smell fresh pie downstairs. Grandmother makes one every morning. Bercaws eat pie the way other folks consume toast.

Before we left Florida on the drive to Virginia, I had overheard my father tell his best friend Joe Dineen that Grandmother had written and was "none too happy" that Beau is divorcing my mother and planning to marry Nora, who works in his office. Grandmother had written of her disapproval.

Dear Beau,

Naturally I have thought of little else since you came up to tell me that you were leaving your family for another woman. It is the saddest thing that has happened in my life. There are several questions I would like to ask that I did not find out when you were here....

What is the cause of Nora's divorce? Is she seeking it, or her husband? It is because of you? What is going to become of their children...?

Her letter troubled Beau deeply, and he told her so. He had also begun calling her "Nana," which is how Lee and I affectionately refer to our grandmother. Usually, Beau addressed his mother by her first name. I had never heard him say "Mom," nor had I ever seen him write it. She had always been Nancy to him, and his father had always been Berc.

Veterans Administration

February 4, 1983

Dear Nana

Your letter to me may be the saddest of all my life and indeed the most hurtful. It doesn't matter though. I've hurt all that I can hurt + survive....

The letter writing began in January and lasted until August. Upon Grandmother's final approval—with the caveat that the lovers sleep in separate rooms—we left for the farm.

Once they marry, Beau and Nora are planning to relocate three hours south of Largo, in Naples, to start all over again with a new neurology practice.

"Kids, get down here!" Beau bellows because he wants to get out on the Rivanna before the midday heat descends. He likes the fact that the size of his family has doubled. Four kids on the farm again, just as it was when he was growing up.

Kathy races downstairs once her swimsuit and shorts are on. I grab the ChapStick from the top of the dresser and stop to look at the two weathered books stacked next to a small blue vase with dried flowers. *The Adventures of Huckleberry Finn* and *Swiss Family Robinson*. I know them both well. Beau had circled these two on my reading list, and put three stars next to each one.

I open up *Huck Finn* and read a paragraph:

> We said there warn't no home like a raft, after all. Other places do seem so cramped up and smothery, but a raft don't. You feel mighty free and easy and comfortable on a raft.

"Gal, come get your breakfast!" Beau is yelling for me again. I shut the book and run downstairs. Grandmother is leaning back in her wicker chair as she always does. Her forefinger rests on the round kitchen table for balance. Craig and Kathy are savoring their fresh warm pie. We work hard, play hard and eat well at the farm.

We had spent the whole first day clearing out the overgrowth down by the river. Beau poured gasoline on the poison ivy. We all took turns firing the shotguns to scare the snakes away. We came back up for a lunch of boiled ham and cabbage, then took long naps before heading back down again to make use of our work.

Lee has finished two pieces of pie by the time I sit down with my slice. Beau is furiously shoving drinks, ice and snacks into a cooler.

"Dagnabit," he says.

"What is it, Beau?" Grandmother asks.

"We've got no Snickers bars."

Grandmother chuckles. She points to the top drawer in the credenza. There was always something sweet in there.

Beau opens the drawer and lets out a sigh of relief. He lifts out a bag of Halloween candy filled with mini Snickers and Three Musketeers.

"Manna from heaven," he says, giggling. "Okay, kids, let's go."

We traipse down the hill—Craig helping Beau with the cooler, Kathy and I carrying the towels and life preservers, Lee toting the big Thermos of homemade lemonade. The canoe, which we had unloaded from the van upon arrival, is waiting for us on the riverbank.

"Gal goes in front with one paddle. I'll take the rear with the other," Beau commands. "Line up by birth order behind Nancy."

Kathy is fourteen. Craig and Lee are both ten. Lee looks at Beau for how to handle the situation.

"Craig is a few months older than you, son."

Lee and I know very little about Kathy and Craig. We had never even met them until a few days ago when Beau told us all to pile into the back of his van. We sat on a mattress in the sweltering heat for eighteen hours, playing Mad Libs and sleeping. You can learn a lot about a person by what nouns, verbs, adjectives, adverbs and body parts they give in Mad Libs. For some reason the word "elbow" made all four of us laugh like crazy. We emerged from the van in Virginia as a family. It was a risky calculation by Beau, but it worked.

Now, Beau uses his paddle to push us in to the middle of the Rivanna. There is an area of rocks and rapid water ahead, but Beau and I had navigated them on many occasions. We pass easily and float for a while, watching cattle graze on the hills. Kathy leads us in a rousing rendition of "99 Bottles of Beer on the Wall."

A few years earlier, Lee and I had been canoeing with Beau in the Myakka River, in central Florida, when we came upon a terrifying situation. We had reached a place where we could no longer put our paddles in the water without hitting an alligator. Lee and I were so frightened we couldn't move a muscle.

"Are we going to die, Dad?" I asked as calmly as I could.

"Not today." He was actually grinning, enlivened by the moment.

Beau told Lee and me to sing "Old Man River" as loudly as we could. I wasn't sure if it was to get our minds off the predators or to help scare the gators away.

Lee and I belted out "he just keeps rolling, he just keeps rolling" over and over again while our father paddled furiously, hitting gators on the snout for leverage. When we tired of the song, Beau instructed us to sing "Way down upon the Suwannee River."

Here on the river with Craig and Kathy, we have very little to fear. There are no gators, just trout, frogs, snakes and turtles. Craig keeps a running count of how many cows we see on the surrounding foothills of the Blue Ridge Mountains. Beau keeps a lookout for snakes. He has brought along a tourniquet just in case one of us gets bit and has to stop the blood flow while he sucks the venom out. Never swallow the venom, he warned, or you'll be dead as a doornail.

"They won't bother us in the boat, though," he says of Rivanna's cottonmouth moccasins. "Usually you see them sunning themselves on the rocks. They scare easily."

Lee suggests that we have a snack. Beau agrees and gives him the high honor of passing out the candy.

Lee reaches around to the cooler, which is in front of Beau, and pulls out the bag. He stands up to hand one toward me, trying to pass it over Craig's and Kathy's heads.

"Buzzard tail, sit down!" Beau yells.

The canoe lists to the left. I try to lean to the right, but it's no use. We capsize. The water is shallow enough that we can all stand. We're safe, but I'm afraid of what my father will do. No one says a word.

Beau starts laughing like a madman. His reaction is so funny, that we all start laughing too. We manage to pull the canoe up on a small sand bar. Then, we roll around in the sand laughing even more. Beau gets the hiccups and some chocolate comes out of his nose.

We dump the water out of the canoe and set off again, only to capsize three more times before we reach the bridge in Columbia. We fall over once because Kathy does a back flip off the boat at Beau's urging. We tip another time because I change places with Craig. And we go over yet again when Craig tries to pee over the edge. The two-hour trip turns into four.

Nora is waiting for us atop the Columbia Bridge, looking upriver for us, her waist-length brown hair flying around in the light breeze. She waves wildly when she sees us.

Beau stands up to wave back. The canoe capsizes again. Nora comes rushing down the riverbank to the little dock. Beau runs through the shallows to embrace her. They're like high-school sweethearts, giddy upon the sight of one another after even the shortest absence.

The way they canoodle reminds me of my first boyfriend, who was "suspect" according to Beau. When Roger called late one night to speak with me, Beau said, "We don't take calls here past 8 p.m.," and hung up on him.

Roger called right back and said it was urgent.

"What could be so urgent to interrupt our evening family time? This better be good, young man."

My boyfriend explained that his mother had just committed suicide. Beau sighed and allowed him to speak with me but "only for three minutes."

Dad stood next to me, holding a small clock, while I tried to think of some fast way to comfort my grieving friend. I told him to read the Bible—a suggestion meant more for my father's ears than my boyfriend's. After we hung up, I begged Beau to let me go see Roger.

"No," he said. "It's bedtime."

"Even though his mom is dead?"

"Lots of people are dead, Gal."

"Mommmmmmmm," Craig screams, bringing me back to the present in the canoe. "I never had more fun, ever!"

"Me either," Kathy yells.

"Or me," says Lee.

I look at Beau who is grinning from ear to ear. Maybe he won't have time to keep fighting what's in his head with all of us around. Maybe he will let go for a while and we'll all float like Huck Finn: *free and easy and comfortable.*

We get back to the farm and head upstairs for naps. I pick up the *Huck Finn* book and take it into the boys' room.

"Craig," I say, "this was Beau's when he was a kid. I think you should have it."

"Thanks, Nan," he says drowsily, tucking it under his arm.

I tell Beau later that I gave the book to Craig.

Beau points to my forehead. "Good thinking, Gal. Good thinking. You're finally using your head for something more than a hat rack."

CHAPTER NINE

ANONA UNITED METHODIST CHURCH

LARGO, FLORIDA

I am eighteen and it is May of 1984—the night before Beau and Nora's wedding. My recurring dream makes another appearance. I have had it a dozen times in the past year—ever since my mother and brother moved away from 310 Harbor View Lane and into a condo near Tampa Bay.

I live in the dorms at the University of South Florida, where Beau is now a professor of neurology with privileges at the James A. Haley Veterans' Hospital. He decided to make a clean break from Largo, where people were whispering about his strange defection from his family. Beau and Nora plan to move to Naples, after he devotes this interim time to teaching neurologists of the future as well as healing soldiers from the past.

In my dream, I am walking someplace and see a head on the ground. At first, I think that someone has been decapitated. But as I get closer I realize the head has two little feet and is walking and talking.

"Hello," I say, looking down at the head, and trying to pretend it's a completely normal situation.

"Hello," he says back. The head is a young man.

"Where are you going?" I ask.

"To school," he says.

"Is it far from here?"

"Nope, just around the corner."

I want to carry him, but he appears fine. He doesn't have a backpack or anything. How could he? He doesn't have arms. I wonder where his stomach and kidneys are. How can he process food for energy? How does he eliminate food? But clearly there is some way because he's alive and seemingly angst-free, unlike me.

"OK, then, have a great day!" I say.

"You, too," says the head, and he trots off.

Then I see a mushroom cloud in the distance. I realize the world is coming to an end. It's a nuclear holocaust. I can feel the wind pick up and I know radioactive material isn't far behind.

I run home—to 310 Harbor View Lane in Largo— where my Civil War signal-tower tree house is, and where Beau has a den filled with neurology books.

I forget about the atomic bomb, which has not come to bear, and pull all of the books down from the shelf. I sit down and start thumbing through one and then another, looking for a picture of a person who is solely composed of a head. I look through two hundred books. I don't stop for anything. I don't eat or drink. I have to find out what's wrong with that boy. I need a name for his condition.

Finally, I find it. But it's not in a neurology textbook or journal. Rather, it's in a freak-show guide that has been stuffed in with the professional literature.

A man named Avuncular stands on top of a high box and crowds look up at him. From this view, they can see that his internal organs are all pushed up into the cranial cavity, sharing space with his brain. It's all there. He has no brain damage, and is quite articulate. He also seems to be very proud of himself. He is smiling. No, he's beaming.

Avuncular knows he is rare. He believes himself to be superior, the caption tells me. But nowhere can I find the name for his condition. Plenty of children have been born with-out heads or brains, but I see no history of body-less babies.

I try to call my father, but my fingers keep slipping off the dial. I lie down on his pink corduroy couch with *Pedi-atric Neurology for the Clinician*.

The phone rings, but I can't get up to answer it. My legs don't work. I'm only four steps from the desk, but it's no use. My legs are paralyzed. I reach around for the spinal-column skeleton hanging from an IV hook. It's on wheels. I use it to slide to the phone. The spinal cord clatters and bangs against me. I pick up the phone and fall to the floor.

"Hello, Dad? Is it you?"

"Hi, is this Nancy?" The voice is not my father's.

"Yes, who is this?" I ask.

"It's Adam, the boy you met earlier today."

"When you were on your way to school?"

"Yes, that's me!"

"How did you get this number?"

"Your dad gave it to me."

I am speechless.

"He wanted me to tell you that I am fine. Please don't worry. I can live like this forever."

"What is the name of your condition?" I ask.

He's answering me, but I can't understand what he's say-ing. His speech is garbled and there's static on the line. I ask him to repeat what he just said.

The line goes dead.

I wake up.

This time, though, I wake up to the realization that my father is getting remarried. I get dressed in the outfit Nora bought for me— a cream-colored shirt, and skirt with multicolored vertical stripes. My brother puts on the suit Beau bought for him. He looks like a young undertaker.

My mother turns on the television. None of us knows what to say. We let the weather reporters do all the talking. It's going to be sunny and humid, with a slight chance of rain in the afternoon. Typical early summer in Florida, although today is anything but typical.

But then again, there has never been a normal day with Beau.

I think about the implications of genetics and divorce. If Beau no longer loves Barbara, does it mean that the Bercaw in me will come to resent the Rixey in me? Am I doomed to self-loathing? I picture Bercaw chromosomes doing a victory dance over Rixey ones. "We're dominant!" they yell, while the Rixey genes recede into oblivion.

I can't believe my father isn't concerned about how difficult it will be for his kids to leave their mother's house to attend his wedding. Or, even if he is, he doesn't acknowledge it. The only thing he told us was to not be late.

Just before we leave, my mother asks if she can brush my hair. We go into her bathroom and I sit on her vanity chair. She starts brushing my long blonde hair.

"Nan, do you remember that brain in a jar in your father's office?"

"Of course I do. It scared the hell out of me. Kind of like dad does."

"That brain belonged to his father."

"What?"

"Yes, that was Berc's brain. Your dad kept it after the autopsy."

I put my head down on the sink. Holy Mother of God. He is insane, obsessed and scared. Or else my mother has lost her mind in a moment of agony over Beau.

"Mom, are you kidding?"

"No, Nan, it's true."

"Why didn't you ever tell me?"

"I don't know, but I thought you needed to know now." An hour before Beau's wedding to another woman, my mother decides to open up.

"Mom, what was Grandfather like?"

"Berc never really knew me or remembered who I was. Beau told me not to get in conversations with him. When I was finishing my master's and pregnant with you in July 1965, I stayed at Rebelanna a couple of weeks. Berc would ask Grandmother, 'What's she doing here?' He also told me not to slam the refrigerator door. He stayed to himself even then, read the paper over and over and asked what day it was over and over. I had to turn off the stove that he left going. Beau had gone on ahead to Air Force Boot Camp. I was sad and sorry for all of us. Of course, it was hardest for your Grandmother."

"What was Berc like before he got sick?" I ask. I keep thinking my quiet, sweet, broken-hearted mother will stop talking. She doesn't.

"Disease or not, I had the impression Berc did not like women. He was against Beau getting married. David and Beau thought he might get up in church and say he had reasonable doubt and stop everything at the last minute. I always thought of him as an angry person. He was proud of his life in the cavalry. He was strict, Southern and literate, though it didn't show in his conversation. He read war books and wrote a lot."

"How did Dad feel about him?"

"Beau seemed to hate his dad, who was known to beat your Grandmother. Berc gave Beau his old Buick when he went to college and also $40,000 worth of Ralston Purina stock to use the dividends to pay his college costs. He made Beau give that back when we got married. I paid for all our living expenses for six years or so. Still, Beau held the loss of the stock over *me*—my fault he lost that stock which might be a fortune now."

Now my docile mother is getting angry and tearful. Yet, she continues. I take the hairbrush out of her hand.

"There was a lot of talk about 'disowning' the four boys. I think it was a threat that meant they would not get an inheritance."

"Mom, what was Beau like as a kid?" I want to get as much out of her as I can before she shuts down.

"He was so brilliant that he skipped second grade. But in third, he couldn't remember if spaces came between words or sentences!"

She laughs at what she's said and then tears up again.

"Beau and I were both survivors in different ways with big troubles in our families in 1965. But I don't know what we could have done. The Vietnam War provided us with an escape to the Philippines."

My mother goes to lie down on the couch to watch *Little House on the Prairie*. Her life hasn't been easy. The day that I was born, her mother died of cirrhosis of the liver at the young age of forty-two. Barb must have spent her youth with a very drunken mom. Her father had dropped dead on the tennis court at Annapolis years before then. My mother's heart was broken long before today.

I want to throw up. I want to run away. But as usual, I do nothing but comply with what Beau has asked of me—what he has trained me to do. I get my brother and go to the wedding in my mother's car. She lets me use it because she knows that Beau hasn't arranged a ride for us.

On the way to Anona Church, it occurs to me that Nora shared my father's world of brains and jars more than we ever did. They bonded over Parkinson's and Alzheimer's and MRI machines and L-dopamine while we busied ourselves with Carlouel Yacht Club and Bible School and the Clearwater Public Library and McDonald's.

The hemispheres of my father's brain had been deeply divided: one side for family; the other side for work. As he got older, and as Berc's dreaded illness started showing up in more and more patients, the work side became more urgent.

Nora brings Beau back to life.

Kathy and Craig meet Lee and me at the church, looking just as tired as we feel. Craig looks a little sadder, though. And Lee looks mad, as if the whole Green Bean Incident is happening all over again.

"How's your dad?" I ask them.

Craig shrugs. Kathy puts her arm around him.

"I had that weird, scary dream again," I tell her. Kathy and I have become good friends. I am glad to have a sister as well as another brother. I marvel at the fact that Beau has found a new wife with kids of similar age and interests. Clones without the tainted Bercaw gene pool.

"The little head?" she asks.

"What does it mean now?" I respond.

"It means our parents are mixing us up. We don't know where we fit. We're that head."

"It's not Beau's head?"

"No," Kathy says. "It represents us four kids, crammed into the back of a van or a canoe."

Maybe she is right, but still I am leaning toward the idea that it's Beau trying to cram so much life into his own skull that everything else gets left out. Maybe us kids are actually the missing limbs. Beau's head is out there on its own—without us.

My dad rushes us to our seats. He talks with the minister, as a handful of other people begin to enter the church.

The organist begins playing "Here Comes the Bride." Everyone stands and turns to the back of the church to watch Nora come down the aisle.

Everyone except me.

I look at my father. I want to see Nora through his eyes. Beau looks up, after saying a silent prayer. The sunlight of the open church doors hits his face. He smiles his big grin, and then he swallows hard. He reaches for the handkerchief in his pocket. He wipes at his eyes. I reach for the tissues my mother suggested I put in my purse. I wipe at my eyes.

Our crying intensifies with every note, and with each step Nora takes toward him in her pretty cream-colored dress. Her long brown hair is up. Both my father and I are weeping as if it were a funeral. Love kills us.

CHAPTER TEN

THE SERENGETI

KENYA, EAST AFRICA

Beau's head is sticking out of the roof of the green vehicle we have used to cover about 500 kilometers of Kenya. Tiny Nora, in the back seat, is engulfed by the huge bags on either side of her. She has proven herself to be just as adventurous as Beau, and I adore her for it.

I have been a Peace Corps volunteer in East Africa for a year. It is 1987. I am twenty-one. Beau and Nora have come to see me and the country. I am proud to share what I have learned with my dad for a change. I am the boss here.

Beau asks me to stop, in the middle of Kenya's backcountry, next to a shack that has a huge sign telling customers to "Pop in for a Coffin." Good thing we didn't actually need a coffin, Beau points out after he's surveyed the area, because there is neither a proprietor nor a coffin on site.

By the time we reach the entrance of the Samburu National Reserve, Beau's face is covered in orange-brown dust. The children in town, who would otherwise rush up to any car and ask for a shilling, keep their distance from the giant red head sticking out of the roof of the green vehicle.

We walk inside the five-star hotel looking like extras from *Raiders of the Lost Ark*. I suspect we smell quite bad, as well.

"Most people come with a safari guide," says the Kenyan desk clerk at the reception desk.

"I am the guide," I tell him in Swahili. "And this man is a chief."

I point at my father, who is wearing a khaki hat that says "Jambo Bwana" which partially covers his dirty face. Grinning wildly from ear to ear, he looks more like a madman than a medicine man.

Nora goes in search of a glass of wine. Her nerves are shot from seven hours of driving on a road so bumpy that we couldn't go faster than fifteen kilometers per hour.

The clerk makes little clicking sounds indicating his mistrust and disinterest in us.

I lift up the stinking Colobus-monkey headdress that the Maragoli people—near Munzatsi Secondary School, where I teach English literature—have given Beau.

"Kuangalia hii!" I say. *Look at this!*

"Please leave all dry cleaning with the valet," the clerk says dismissively.

Beau laughs so hard he nearly falls down. He loves the fact that we have switched Colonial race-roles with the Kenyan. I love this side of my father. Recalcitrance.

"Gal, tell him we have six sheepskins in the Jeep that need cleaning too."

"Sir, I speak English," the clerk snaps, growing weary of the dirty white Bercaws and their antics. "Here are your room keys. Dinner is served at 7 p.m. Jackets and ties are required for gentlemen. If you don't have one, we can supply one for you."

"Guess you can't wear your headdress, Dad."

Beau is doubled over at this point, tears turning his face into a mud pie. He looks like the landscape we just traversed. En route to the resort, we had tried to cross a small river in the Jeep and gotten stuck in the mud. Nora took the wheel while Beau and I pushed. The rear tires sprayed dirty water on us like a hose. I told Beau and Nora that we had no time to waste because these waters, even the shallow ones, were home to crocodiles that made Florida alligators look like kittens.

Now in the hotel, we find our rooms with the help of several porters, who struggle with our unwieldy luggage and unlikely souvenirs. We had been on the move for two weeks, and this is our last stop.

I had picked this location because it was where George and Joy Adamson had lived with their lioness Elsa. I first heard about the couple while watching *Born Free* on Disney with Beau. On that one and only occasion, he had let me continue watching the movie even though it went an hour past my bedtime.

"One day, Daddy, I'll go there," I'd said back then. "I swear to God."

"Don't swear, Gal," Beau chastised me. "God doesn't like it. If you want to go, just go. But, of course, you have to take me."

Our first stop on this trip had been at the Maasai Mara Reserve. We flew from Nairobi on a small bush plane. I wanted to start there because we could take a hot air balloon ride over the Serengeti and stay in tented camps that were as elegant as any Ritz Carlton. I figured we would get more rustic as the trip unfolded.

After dinner that first night, we couldn't get back to our tents because a herd of zebra were in the way. All of our white-gloved African waiters had to leave the dining room and go shush the zebras aside.

Beau said, "This is a real life Rorschach test. What do you see when black Africans in white gloves are herding black-and-white-striped zebra?"

"Whirling dervishes," I said.

"To me, it looks like the zigzags of an EKG," Beau said.

Nora said, "All I can see are two crazy Bercaws."

The morning of our balloon flight was unusually windy, especially for 5 a.m. The driver took us to the flat plain on the Mara where we would embark once the wind calmed down. When it finally did, we rushed into the giant basket. But just as we got inside, a huge gust pulled the balloon along the ground and brush for a few hundred yards before the pilot made the decision to ascend quickly.

There were six of us in the balloon: Beau, Nora, me, the pilot and another American couple—one of whom complained about her ankle the entire time we floated above herds of water buffalo and giraffe. I could tell my father was annoyed that she was calling attention to herself instead of admiring the landscape, which was even more beautiful than it had appeared in *Out of Africa*.

Our descent was less exciting, and back on the ground we were greeted with a champagne breakfast. Even after a few sips, hurt-ankle lady was still whining.

"Let me see that thing," Beau snapped, pushing his caviar away. "I'm a doctor."

He examined the foot, swigging champagne, and declared the woman a "first-class wimp" and "el stupido for wearing high heels on a hot air balloon safari."

She was speechless. Her husband helped her hobble over to the minivan and demanded that the driver take them back to the Camp. Beau, Nora and I stayed put, enjoying the champagne and adrenaline high at 7 a.m. in the very place where mankind crawled out of the Great Rift Valley. A guard stayed behind to keep us safe from lions, with nothing but a spear.

Later that evening, the manager of Governors' Camp told Beau that the woman had been taken to the hospital in Nairobi and was undergoing surgery. Beau just laughed and said, "Serves her right."

The manager had more champagne sent to our tents. He was grateful that Beau would probably defend Governors' Camp if ankle-lady tried to sue for being injured on the balloon's bumpy takeoff.

We flew back to Nairobi after five days of animal-watching in complete luxury. I warned Beau and Nora that our trip was about to get a lot more rustic. Beau clapped and said, "Yeeeehaaaaaawww!"

I rented the green Jeep in Nairobi and we headed for my school —about 250 kilometers west, near Lake Victoria. Beau and his Rotary Club had donated enough money to help the Munzatsi School build a library and to stock it with a few hundred books. My father and Nora timed their trip to coincide with the library's grand opening.

When we pulled into the school's gates, the students greeted us by singing and dancing. The headmaster shook my father's hand for five minutes straight and then escorted us to a blanket under one of the largest acacia trees in the school compound. The local mamas in colorful kikoys delivered hot tea, warm beer, toasted bread and hard-boiled eggs on huge trays balanced on their heads.

"The food is cooked and will be safe," I whispered in my father's ear. "But the cups and dishes were probably washed in cold water. The Maragolis don't have access to clean water. I boil mine."

My father whispered back, "Gandhi said it's better to get sick than to insult your hosts."

I nodded to the headmaster who presented my father with the Maragoli homebrew in a teacup.

"Between the high-octane beer and the possible *E.coli*," I whispered to Nora. "Beau could be in for major stomach issues. Did he bring antibiotics?"

She nodded.

Dozens of bare-footed students gathered around us in their uniforms of turquoise shirts and brown shorts. They sang the Kenyan national anthem and a few tribal hymns before being dismissed by the headmaster to the dirt basketball court.

The mamas and the other teachers also retreated to make way for five male Maragoli tribal elders, dressed in bright wraps and sandals made from old tires. They had walked for miles to meet my father. The *mzee*, Swahili for eldest, sat next to Beau and presented him with the Colobus-monkey headdress, as well as a hand-carved stool and a tribal spear. The other elders helped Beau onto the stool and put the headdress on him. They spoke mainly in Maragoli—the people and their language sharing the same name—so I had no idea what they were saying. I figured that this was the inaugural time any white man had been part of such a ceremony because a common Swahili word, "kwanza," which means first, was being tossed around too.

The elders and the chief walked Beau to the new structure. The headmaster pointed to a plaque on the door that said "*Bercaw Library.*"

Beau threw his arms up into the air. The tribal members followed suit, and then the headmaster, the teachers, the mamas and the students did so as well. Nora and I shrugged and then raised our arms too. There we were: two hundred people—three of them white—standing in very rural Kenya next to Bercaw Library with our hands in the air.

The headmaster broke the silence with the announcement—first in English, then in Maragoli—that a feast was being prepared at his home. The Bercaws and the chief were the honored guests. A lamb would be sacrificed.

Lamb?

I had lived in Kenya for nearly a year and had never seen a lamb sacrificed. Goats and chickens yes, but not a lamb. The Maragolis were the poorest of the poor, how could they afford to give one up?

And, unknowingly, to the man who once stopped my 12th grade teacher from letting us dissect the brain of one. I had informed Beau that we would be dissecting a lamb's brain in Anatomy and Physiology the next day, and he calmly asked for the name of my teacher and looked her up in the Largo White Pages.

"Mrs. Andrews, this is Dr. Bercaw. Your class will not be dissecting lamb brains tomorrow or any other day. The nervous system of lambs carries a fatal disease called scrapie, a transmissible spongiform encephalopathy. Thank you and have a nice evening."

"What did she say, Dad?"

"Nothing. I hung up after I gave her the information."

I shrugged. Beau perceived my reaction as smug, disinterested. I watched his expression shift into rage.

"Know what happens when you get scrapie or Creutzfeldt-Jakob Disease? Imagine Parkinson's and *ALZ-HEIM-ER'S* put together. Muscle spasms, lack of muscle control, and memory loss until your mind and body shrivel up and die. Nothing to take lightly, Gal."

The way he said Alzheimer's, emphasizing each syllable with such vengeance, took my breath way.

What would Beau do now? Break Gandhi's rule and risk getting scrapie? We had no idea how the lamb was going to be cooked, or which parts, for that matter.

I held my breath.

Beau looked at me. His eyes said *fix it.*

"Headmaster," I said, "it is my father's wish that he provide the meal this evening. He is the one who is honored to be a Maragoli now and must offer a sacrifice of his own. He would like to have the feast here at the school for everyone and to pay for all the food."

"As he wishes."

I took three students aside, and gave them money to buy enough chickens and goats to feed the crowd. I told the mamas to bring more tea, bread and eggs. I gave the headmaster some cash as a token of my father's appreciation.

I announced that the mzungu *(white)* Maragoli chief needed to rest. We would return when the sun had set and the meal was ready. I quietly instructed Beau to give all his shillings to the elder chief for beer.

We got in the Jeep and headed for the Sunset Hotel in Kisumu with no intention of returning to the school that evening. But it wouldn't matter anyway, because everyone would be full, drunk and forever grateful to my father. By morning, the headmaster would be writing to him for more money. And my father, no doubt, would send it.

The day after that, we had set off for the Mount Kenya Safari Club, the most regal and elegant hotel in Kenya, located at the base of Mount Kenya. We wandered the gardens by day and sat by the fireplaces in our rooms by night. Over one of our five-course dinners, I asked Beau if he had ever been to a finer hotel.

"Maybe the Lake Palace in Rajasthan, India," he answered. "But the YMCA in New Delhi is perfectly decent. You should see Asia next, Gal."

"What about the Royal Hotel in Nepal?" I countered. "Was that the best place ever?"

"No, this is better," he said.

"Raffles in Singapore?"

Beau shook his head, indicating that the time for questions was over. Truth was that my dad was as happy in a diner as he was in a five-star hotel.

After we had left the Safari Club, and headed north to our final destination, Samburu Land, we happened upon a police checkpoint.

"Dad, all they want is baksheesh. Bribe money. Let me do the talking."

Beau opened up the moon roof of the Jeep and stuck his head out to watch. The police officer walked toward our vehicle before stopping in his tracks. The sight of a huge white man emerging from the top of a Jeep startled him.

I stood up on my seat and poked my head out of the hatch too. *"Bwana, mzee ni daktari. Na, mzee ni mafuo kubwa kitika kichwa."* The police officer waved us on.

"Gal did it!" Beau hollers down to Nora. "She beat the *polisi* at their own game!"

I sat back down to drive. Beau stayed in his upright position—enjoying the view.

"What did you say to them?" Nora asked me.

"This man is a doctor," I told her. "*And* he is sick in the head." Nora laughed.

"There is nothing that Kenyans fear more than something being wrong with their brain," I told her. "I guess that makes them honorary Bercaws."

Beau kept his head out of the Jeep for the next six hours, all the way to the Samburu Serena Safari Lodge.

He sat down once to ask me if there were cannibals in Kenya.

"Dad," I answered. "If so, they aren't gonna eat you. That's for damn sure."

CHAPTER ELEVEN

THE 38TH PARALLEL

SOUTH KOREA

I am in a staring contest with a North Korean soldier. It is 1988 and I am twenty-three. We are about three feet apart, separated by the DMZ and a chain-link fence. I feel much the way I did when Beau and I were behind the fence at the public pool in Alabama. All I want to do is cross over and see what happens. I wish my father were here to test the waters with me, but he is embroiled in his own stalemate back in Naples, Florida.

I had come to South Korea to teach English at a private language school and watch the 1988 Summer Olympics in person, especially the swimming events. My archrival in college turned into the fastest sprinter in America and was on the U.S. team. My career had ended with a bad shoulder, and surgery. I was ready to define myself outside the water and away from my father, a journey I had begun in Kenya.

I also chose Korea because my uncle Woodson had served here during the Korean War—right where I'm standing at the 38th Parallel. Berc helped in this war effort too, but from Washington, D.C.

When I blink, the soldier opposite me blinks. When I squint, he squints. If I sigh, he does. He is mirroring me. If the USO tour guide hadn't informed me that the North Korean was likely to do so, I would think the soldier suffered from a neurological condition, called echopraxia—a symptom of Tourette's syndrome in which those affected feel an uncontrollable urge to mimic an action after seeing it being performed. Beau taught me all sorts of neurological facts. I had been his apprentice.

If my father were here, he would surreptitiously turn this "war game" into a neurological evaluation—studying the North Korean soldier for any indications of damage to his frontal lobe. My father is adroit at reading symptoms, syndromes and scans. He is a master diagnostician. He is always sizing people up—looking for signs of weakness in their systems, and sometimes in their souls.

Before I came to South Korea, I had overheard my father talking to one of his colleagues about Down syndrome increasing the chances of getting early-onset Alzheimer's by three to five times. The comment made me wonder if Bercaws passed down some variation of an unknown chromosome—a previously unheard of phenomenon characterized by antisocial, obsessive-compulsive behavior, as well as strange physical traits such as towering height, big lips on strong jaws, and weak joints. Bercaw syndrome led to one outcome: an atrophied brain just as in Alzheimer's. Maybe our brains actually diminish from overuse and fixation, as if they have no choice but to recoil from our recurring thoughts.

This North Korean and I have more in common than our coordinated movements. Besides the fact that MacArthur played a role in each of our histories, I see similarities in our forefathers: Kim Il Sung and Grandfather Berc. Two tyrants. I wish I could tell the soldier what I am thinking, but Army personnel warned me that talking could get me shot. Silence and guns rule in North Korea, just as they do in every Bercaw household.

On the other side of the world, my father is locked in his own Cold War. I had called him a week earlier from my small apartment in Seoul. I needed comfort, or possibly I needed him to worry.

"Dad, a friend of mine was murdered in her sleep. I'm sad and I'm scared.

"I feel like the South Koreans are turning against Americans now too. It's like they've forgotten that we liberated them from the Japanese."

I told Beau how the students to whom I was teaching English were spending their days protesting the American military presence in Seoul. They brought their tear gas masks to class. They didn't seem to find it incongruous that they wanted to get rid of Americans in Korea, and yet wanted to visit America themselves. And now, my friend had been killed in her bed—stabbed head to heel and ear to ear. Her death was all over the newspapers and television.

The Korean Police believed an American had killed her. Meanwhile, our American teaching staff was sure that the crime had been committed by a Korean. I recounted all this to my father, as quickly as I could, so he wouldn't interrupt.

Beau was silent on the other end for a long time. Finally, he responded.

"Gal, welcome to the real world. People get murdered every day. Wars come and go. It's all cyclical. Now listen to me, Gal, listen to what I have to deal with here."

Beau was in fierce battle with Naples Community Hospital. He launched into a tirade of epic proportions, complete with imitations of the parties involved. He was uncharacteristically animated.

"Gal, those goddamned lawyers challenged my integrity."

"Dad, I feel like the whole country of Korea is doing that to me."

"Gal, listen to what I am telling you. I am suing Naples Community Hospital for antitrust. They only want to pay the radiologists for reading the MRIs. It's not right. Radiology is a made-up profession. I am the Sherlock Holmes of brain scans. I find clues in MRI scans that no one else can. They should pay me to do my work. I'm going to look at the scans anyway."

"Maybe, Dad, you should bring your Sherlock Holmes skills here and solve the mystery of my friend's murder."

He didn't hear me, or more likely, he ignored me.

"The hospital and the Board of Trustees don't understand that I have devoted my working life to studying the brain. I bought the first CT scanner in the State of Florida with my own money. I was a leading proponent of the MRI machine because it sees inside my patients' heads without opening them up. It saves time, money and lives. Furthermore, I have taken every imaging course in existence."

"Dad, I'm sorry you have to go through that. Are you going to win the case?"

"I'd better. It's costing me a fortune to make a point."

"The FBI is looking into the murder of my friend," I countered. "We're all going to be questioned. I suppose I will have to appear in court sometime to testify on her character."

"Character is everything, Gal. That's what is killing me about this situation here. Naples Community Hospital lacks character. They need to understand what is right and what is wrong."

"And you are going to teach them?"

"Remember the Fat Albert TV cartoon? How he always learned a lesson at the end of a show?"

"So, you're giving NCH their Fat Albert lesson?"

"Someone has to, Gal."

And with that, my father hangs up the phone. He doesn't say "goodbye" or "your ol' dad sure loves you."

He had said all he wanted. Meanwhile, somewhere else in the United States, the father of my beautiful dead friend was grieving his daughter. I guess I had hoped that my dad would want to solve this case as if it were a medical mystery. But Beau's message was always the same: life is full of death. There is no cure.

CHAPTER TWELVE

CLARK AIR BASE

THE PHILIPPINES

"Welcome home!" says the Filipino immigration agent when he notices the place of birth in my passport. After a year of saving every penny in frozen Korea, I arrive in steamy Manila in the spring of 1989. I'll be twenty-four in December and I hope to learn something about my fifty-one-year-old father in this country.

After dropping my bags at a guesthouse, I walk the length of the city—from Malacañan Palace, where Imelda Marcos' shoe collection is preserved, to the sex shops in the Makati Pasay Road bar district. I buy a Coke in a McDonald's, which is guarded by a soldier with a machine gun. I nap on a bench in the huge Rizal Park.

Beau, are you here? I ask myself before drifting off.

The next day, I take a bus to Baguio through the winding mountains. I throw up out the window from motion sickness like some of the other Filipino passengers. I arrive in the cooler hill station, as the British once called it, and lie down on the grass. I look up at the sky.

I try to see if I can spot shapes in the cloud puffs. Beau and I used to play this game while lying on the lawn at the old farm. He once offered me $200 if I could find a series of clouds that looked like Ankgor Wat. Best I could do was the Great Wall of China. My dad gave me $10 for the effort.

Once the nausea passes, I walk down Asin Road, where the famed

Baguio furniture-makers congregate to sell their wares. This is where my father had an enormous desk constructed out of indigenous ka-magong wood. Made to his specifications, it accommodated his great height and held his piles of journals, files, paperwork, reflex hammers and prescription pads. Then he placed his father's brain, in a jar, at the center of that universe.

I find a very old Filipino craftsman and watch as he carves the outline of a bird into a serving tray with a small, sharp knife.

"Excuse me," I say.

"Yes?" He gets up from his cross-legged position. He is about half my size. "Are you looking for something special?"

"Were you here in 1965?"

"Yes, I came from Hapao that year. Before Baguio, I carved wood in the forest."

"Do you remember seeing a man who looked like me? A huge, giant man with a big grin and wild blue eyes? An American man who believed he was a Filipino too?"

I sound like I am tracking down a fairy tale. I am.

The old man shakes his head. "I have seen too many people in my life."

"He had a huge desk made somewhere around here. The biggest desk I have ever seen."

"No," he says again, and sits back down to continue his work. He seems disappointed that I'm not going to buy anything. Then he looks up at me again.

"What are you looking for?"

"My father."

"Where is he buried?"

"He's still alive."

"Where?"

"In the United States."

"Why don't you go see him there?"

"Because this is where he was born, and I was too. Part of us is here. But I'm not sure which part."

The carver thinks while he plays with the chair he is working on.

"Go see Dominican Hill. Great view of Baguio up there."

I give him a handful of pesos and head back to town. I ask a cab driver to take me to the top of the hill.

"It's closed," protests the driver. "No more tourists can go there. Not safe. Headless ghosts."

"What?" I ask.

"Diplomat Hotel is there, used to be a seminary. Back in the War, the Japanese turned it into a POW camp. Beheaded nuns and priests inside. Killed babies by the fountain. Very bad place. Filipinos don't go there now."

"Will you drive me past it?" I plead.

"For double money. I play radio loud so we don't hear the screams."

"Screams?"

"Filipinos hear the screams of the dead coming from there."

"When was the hotel in operation?"

"Filipino faith healer bought it in 1973. People came from Europe to be cured in the hotel. He died three years ago. Hotel closed. Bad place."

I'm certain my father would have come to see this place—before it was a hotel—while visiting Baguio.

"Take me as close as you can," I say. "By the way, I was born in the Philippines. My father was too. Maybe I can hear the screams."

"You are a big, white, beautiful Filipina," he says, and chuckles, before hitting the gas. "But crazy one!"

"You should see my dad! Bigger and crazier!"

"What does he do?" the driver asks.

"He's a faith healer," I say.

The driver slows as we approach the old Diplomat Hotel. He turns the radio volume up as high as it will go. It is crackly but I can make out some lyrics. I realize it's the national anthem.

Philippines! My country, my homeland…

Land of mine! In fetters kept,
You suffered as we wept.

"There!" the driver yelps and points toward the old gates.

"Daaaaaaaaaddddddddd!" I yell out the window. "I miiiiiiiissssssssss yoooouuuuu!"

The driver peels out and heads back down the hill. He drops me at a little guesthouse run by his cousin, where I get a room for $5.

I crawl into my tiny bed and fall asleep. When I wake up, a cup of coffee and a slice of toast are waiting on my nightstand.

"I love you Philippines," I say out loud. "You're a whole country of Bercaws afraid of dead people haunting their minds."

I make my way back to the bus station and take the next one bound for Angeles City, home to Clark Air Base. I sit next to the only other Western person onboard. He's a middle-aged British man, who has come to tour World War II sites. He talks with me about the Bataan Death March.

"The Japanese forced 75,000 American and Filipino prisoners to walk for 60 kilometers in the searing heat—with no water or food—and intermittently assaulted them with knives and bayonets. During the three-day march, one quarter of the prisoners died or was killed."

"My dad told me about this. He also said the Americans were so focused on Hitler's crimes that the Japanese atrocities were virtually unknown by people in the West."

"Your dad was right."

"Where did the march take place?" I ask.

"Out there," he points at the window. "Not far from here. This is the province of Pampanga."

"Did they go near Clark?"

"Walked right past the gates. Clark Field was later turned into a concentration camp. The Japanese were flying kamikaze missions out of Clark then."

"I was born at Clark," I tell the British man.

"History is a burden," he sighs. "Or a blessing. Or both."

"I know."

We pull into the bus station in Angeles City, four hours after leaving Baguio.

"What do you think of Americans?" I ask my new friend as we part ways. I don't know why I ask this question. I no longer know why I do anything. I just want my dad to love me, but he is too busy saving brains. And I am here, 9,000 miles away, trying to understand him and his father before him. Beau always used to tell me that "the Philippines are in our blood," so I am hoping that my father will run through me while I'm here.

The British man giggles at my questions. "I like them, but they say 'I love you' too much. Nothing left a mystery for you Yanks." He winks at me. I laugh because he doesn't know my family, in which everything is a mystery.

I consider his comment as I walk in the direction of Clark. His pronouncement, if correct, is further proof that my father is a Filipino, not an American. Beau never said "I love you" to me. It was always in the third person. "Your ol' dad sure loves you." Sometimes I wanted to yell back, "Who is my ol' dad? And where I can find him?"

Beau treated love like a research project. Before I turned thirteen, he sat me down to explain the different kinds of love to me. Instead of the birds-and-bees talk, I got a lecture on C.S. Lewis and ancient Greek.

"There are four kinds of love, Gal. *Eros* is the kind people tend to think of first. It's desire and longing, but it's not everything. There's also *storge*, which is love for your family. And *philia*, which is friendship. Finally, there's *agape*, which is the greatest of all—like God's love for us, caring no matter what the circumstance. You want a relationship that has some of each kind of love."

Beau also taught me how to perform a tracheotomy when we were camping in the El Yunque Rainforest in Puerto Rico when I was nine, so I could save someone I love from dying. I had simply informed my father that he was snoring when he launched into a master course of first aid.

"I must have sleep apnea," he said, pulling out his Swiss Army knife to show me what to do in case he stopped breathing—how to slit his throat just so. "Don't be afraid, Gal. Even if you mess up, it's better than doing nothing while I die."

I find a guesthouse in Angeles City, a mile from the entrance to Clark. I put my backpack down in my tiny, un-air-conditioned room and get my birth certificate out of my wallet.

Place of birth: Angeles City, Pampanga, Philippines. A place where so many Americans and Filipinos died in World War II; a place where my ol' dad tried to save American and Vietnamese servicemen during the Vietnam War. Can I save him from here?

I walk back into the wide streets of Angeles City. Shops line each side, selling T-shirts, Bud Light and sex. I step into one to buy a postcard. I choose a wide-angle vintage picture of the entrance to Clark. I borrow a pen to write.

Dear Dad,

I'm in Angeles City after a day and night of ghost-hunting in Baguio. I've been learning about the Death March. I imagine you here, 30 years ago, trying to stop death in its tracks. I'm not sure we can stop death when it's full-steam ahead like a freight train. It chooses us and we can't outrun it. Maybe war is trying to tell us to stop fighting. Just live in peace until the end comes. By the way, I LOVE YOU OL' DAD. I'll be home soon. I'll go to India first, and then I'll be back.
Love,
Gal

I buy a stamp from the proprietress and she offers to mail the postcard for me. I give her the card.

"How do you say 'thank you' in Tagalog?" I ask.

"*Salamat.*"

"How do you say, 'I love you'?"

She laughs. "We have a lot of ways to say that, but the most common is *'mahal kita.'*"

"Can I have the card back?"

She hands it to me.

I write "P.S. MAHAL KITA."

"You'd make a good Filipino!" the shopkeeper giggles.

Yet, I'm a bad Bercaw for saying how I feel. I should just soldier on in silence on our family's very own Death March. But this one isn't between the Japanese and the Americans and Filipinos.

This is Alzheimer's versus Bercaws.

CHAPTER THIRTEEN

HOTEL YAK AND YETI

KATMANDU, NEPAL

Off and on, for two days, I have been throwing up into a bathtub while I sit on a toilet, tormented by diarrhea, in my hotel room in Kathmandu. When my fever spikes, I imagine that my father is on his way to get me. He is in a medical helicopter coming through the Himalayas. He will set up a MASH unit in the center square and hook up an IV to rehydrate me.

My father was here in 1966. He and my mother had left me in the Philippines under the care of my nanny Veronica when I was only one year old.

How does a parent leave an infant to travel thousands of miles away? I can't think about it or I will vomit again. He was twenty-eight then. I am twenty-four now. It is the summer of 1989 and I wonder if this is when and where my life will end.

Beau warned me of this before I went to Africa. He had given me a list of everything that could cause me to lose my faculties: malaria, typhus, typhoid, schistosomiasis.

"Avoid these illnesses at all costs, Gal," he warned. Was he more concerned about the confusion that might come from a fever than these life-threatening illnesses? Not thinking clearly posed the greatest threat to mankind.

When my fever breaks, I realize I need to find a way to the hospital. There is no phone, so I can't call my father. He would just tell me to find a doctor anyway. I put my jeans on and they fall off. I have been traveling for two months in Asia and have lost twenty pounds. I look like Beau when he was here—stricken with stomach issues and a sinus headache so bad that he bought narcotics from hippies in the street to alleviate his suffering. But I need antibiotics, not heroin. Beau had walked amongst "the drug-addled draft dodgers" in Kathmandu, as he recounted to me on several occasions, because his head hurt so badly and he knew that local poppies offered the only relief in town.

I walk down the stairs, only to have to turn around and run to my bathroom. *How I am going to get to the hospital like this? Dad, help me.*

I put on two pairs of underwear in case I have another blowout. Maybe I can make it to the hospital without poop streaming down my legs. I think of what my cousin said about Grandfather Berc—how he wiped poop on the walls of the farmhouse. *Do I have early onset Alzheimer's?*

I walk out the front of the hotel and wave a rickshaw over.

"To doctor," I say. "Go fast."

The Nepalese are clearly used to taking Western visitors to doctors. The driver gets me to a small clinic in minutes. An American doctor sees me immediately.

"Describe your symptoms," he says.

"I feel like all my organs are crushing in."

"You probably have altitude sickness and amoebic dysentery. Take these for seven days. I'll give you a shot to get the meds flowing."

"I'll live?"

"You'll feel better very soon. Try to drink some water. Bottled water."

"Thank you, doctor. I love you."

He laughs. "I get that a lot."

"One more thing."

"Yes?"

"Could this be signs of dementia to come?"

Because growing up with Beau had been disorienting—I was never certain of where I stood back then—I worry that I may now be experiencing long-term effects. Maybe Beau had created an Alzheimer's disease where there was none.

"No, I think you are hallucinating."

He gives me the shot.

My rickshaw driver is waiting for me, even though I hadn't asked him. He knows I'll need a ride home. Smart Sherpas, always helping white misfits in their country. I already feel better—people are taking care of me.

"Take me to Hotel Yak and Yeti, please," I say. I want to see the reason my father and mother came here in 1966 on their way to India.

India had much more to offer: the Taj Mahal, Jaipur, the Lake Palace.

The only people going to Nepal back then were hippies and climbers. Nepal was north of India, traveling between the two places wasn't easy or quick. So why was Beau so hell-bent on seeing Kathmandu?

He wanted to meet Boris Lissanevitch, the famed exiled Russian who became a ballet dancer in Paris, then a club owner in Calcutta, then a pal of the Nepalese king, then a tiger hunter. Boris opened the Yak and Yeti Bar and Restaurant, as well as the Royal Hotel. Essentially, he opened Nepal to the world.

Beau wrote to Boris, from the Philippines, asking if he could come meet him and to stay at the Royal. Boris wrote back in the affirmative, but with a stipulation.

"Bring a case of Scotch."

My father managed to smuggle only one bottle of Scotch into the still-very-unknown country. After paying this fee, Beau was able to listen to Boris tell stories at the Yak and Yeti bar.

I get out of the rickshaw and ask the doorman if I can use the bathroom.

I throw up in a marble-floored stall of the hotel. There are pictures of mountaineers and their Sherpas on every wall. But more importantly, at least according to Beau, this place is named in honor of the Yeti—Bigfoot's white cousin. I suspect that Beau came here to track him, as well as Boris.

Beau told Lee and me about the mythical creature around our campfire on one occasion. It sounded like the Yeti was a long lost Bercaw. But that was because Beau was making up the story as he went along.

"The Yeti wanders the mountains of Tibet and Nepal alone. He needs no companionship, only food. He'll have eternal life if he can remain unknown to mankind. If he is caught, then he will die. But his territory is being increasingly invaded by climbers. It's getting harder and harder to go unnoticed. Ugly, pink men in bright clothes are everywhere these days, barking orders at small, brown men in rags. The pink men disgust the Yeti. He knows the brown men. They are Buddhists, like him. They will bring him no harm. The pink men are the threat. They will enslave him, the way they do the brown men. The Yeti has to run now. Run to the roof of the world. Get lost in the Pamir Mountains. But one of the pink men has seen his tracks. He is following him. The pink man won't give up. He walks for days and days. The Yeti believes that soon he will have to fight the pink man. The war is coming."

"No, Daddy," I cried in the middle of his story. "The Yeti has to hide. The pink man will kill him. He has weapons."

My father is indifferent to my worry.

"The Yeti finds a cave at the top of K2. The very mountain itself has killed sixty-six men who dared to climb her ragged cliffs and endure her brutal climate. The Yeti is safe here until the pink man can invent a way to survive in his element. That will be a long, long time. Happy at the top of the earth, alone with his own thoughts."

"No other creature to love?" I had asked. My brother stared at my father in disbelief.

"The Yeti doesn't want love. He wants to live. He can't have both."

I put my head on my knees and let out a long wail.

"Gal, let me show you how to do it. This is the way you call the Yeti." My father tilted his head back and howled. "OOOHHHH-HOOOOOHHOOOOOAAAAHHHHO."

Lee ran into the tent. I chased after him and we got in the same sleeping bag, zipping it up all the way. Beau stayed by the fire practicing his yeti call.

"OOHHHHOOOOOHHOOOOOAAAAHHHHO."

I heard a car pull into our site and saw the headlights through the tent. The car door opened and closed.

"Everything OK here, sir?" It was the camp's night manager.

"Just fine," Beau said. "Children thought they saw Bigfoot, and screamed. I might have hollered a bit myself."

"Probably just a coyote," the man said. "Shadows from the fire, that sort of thing."

"Or maybe it was Bigfoot," my dad countered. "There is that possibility."

I heard the car door open and close again. The guy was leaving.

Lee told me he was scared. I started singing, "Yes, Jesus loves me" to him.

Beau came in and joined in the song. "The Bible tells me so."

On my way out of the Yak and Yeti, I stop at the reception desk and ask if I can make a collect call to the United States. The Nepalese clerk points to a room down the hall.

"Go in there and pick up the phone. Tell the operator the number you want to call and that the charges will be reversed."

I give the operator the number for my dad's office. He would be just starting his day. Hopefully I can catch him between patients. The line is ringing. Someone picks up.

"Dr. Bercaw's office."

"Collect call from Nancy Bercaw in Nepal. Do you accept the charges?"

"This is the answering service, I can't accept collect calls. Dr. Bercaw is at the hospital on rounds."

I hang up. My father is busy helping other people.

I ask the registration clerk if Boris still hangs around the hotel.

"He's dead," she answers.

"When?"

"In 1986. Three years ago."

The rickshaw driver is waiting for me. He helps me climb back in the seat and takes me back to my hotel. I fall asleep and wake up feeling better. I take my pill, and walk around a shiny Hindu temple covered with mean little monkeys. The huge eyes on the temple stare down at me.

"What are you looking at?" I want to say. "I'm well aware of the fact that what I'm looking for isn't here."

Ever since I had first heard about Edmund Hillary and the Sherpas, I wanted to climb Everest myself. When I told my father, he said, "You'd do better swimming the English Channel, you wouldn't survive a minute on Everest. You are a child of the tropics."

He was right. I am barely surviving Kathmandu.

After five days, I am well enough to leave Nepal for India, although I'm running out of money. I buy a bus ticket to the border of the two countries, and a train ticket to Delhi from there. This will be a two-day trip overland.

The bus maneuvers down the lush green steppes of the Himalayas at breakneck pace. Sometimes there is only a foot between the bus tires and the drop-off. I can see old rusting smashed-up buses at the bottom of ravines thousands of feet below. I am grateful there aren't any fresh bodies strewn about too. I try to distract myself with the chickens and children on the bus.

I know what Beau would say about this trip. "Gal, more people die on the buses in Nepal than by climbing Everest."

Eight hours later, we reach the border with India. But I am told the train will not be running that night. I need a place to sleep. There is a shabby cement building with "Rooms" painted in red on the side. I knock.

A young woman shows me to one of her rooms. It has a wooden slab for a bed in the middle with a bare light bulb dangling over it.

"One dollar," she says. I give it to her and lie down. I feel like a cadaver in a morgue, but without a blanket to cover my pale boney torso.

I sleep until the next afternoon and then make my way back to the train station for the night ride to Delhi, along with about a thousand other people. I upgrade to a sleeping car by trading the watch my father had given me for college graduation. I want to be comfortable more than I want a Seiko. Beau had traded his Rolex for a carpet here many years ago. I am sure he would understand. Besides, I need what's left of my cash to get to the Taj Mahal.

I wake up just as the sun is rising. The countryside is dotted with people already. I can't tell what they are doing. As the light gets brighter, I realize that they are relieving themselves in the fields. One big latrine as far as the eye can see.

"You do not know suffering, Gal, until you see India," my father once said when I went with him to the Veteran's hospital in Tampa. I had recoiled at the sight of a man's head that was encircled with big stitches that seemed to be holding his cranium in place. My father looked at me with rage. "At least he's alive and in America. He's lucky, you ol' buzzard tail. Get that through your thick skull."

The train arrives in Delhi. A dozen amputee beggars greet us. I take a cab to the YMCA, which my father had highly recommended from his time here in the 1960s.

"Safest place in the city. And spotless," he told me.

I ask the doorman for the best way to get to Agra and the Taj Mahal.

"You need a driver."

"I can't take a bus?"

"No, for safety, you must have a driver."

"Safety from what?" I ask. I'm not afraid of anything except a man who isn't here.

"Too many people wanting things from you."

"I have nothing."

"You have more than them, madam."

"Can you arrange a driver for me? A cheap one?"

"Yes, madam."

Six hours later I am standing in front of the greatest monument to love ever created. Emperor Shah Jahan constructed the Taj in memory of his beloved third wife Mumtaz Mahal, with whom he fell in love at first sight. She died giving birth to their fourteenth child at age thirty-eight.

"There is nothing more beautiful in the world than the Taj Mahal," my father told me long ago. "Except the love Shah Jahan had for Mumtaz. Only that was greater. You will find redemption just by gazing upon the Taj."

The promise was so great that my father had come twice over the course of two decades with two different wives. He had given me the Fodor's guidebook that he used on both trips. A quote from Shah Jahan about the Taj was highlighted in yellow, the same way Beau marked his neurology journals when he needed to remember something important.

> Should guilty seek asylum here,
> Like one pardoned, he becomes free from sin.
> Should a sinner make his way to this mansion,
> All his past sins are to be washed away.
> The sight of this mansion creates sorrowing sighs;
> And the sun and the moon shed tears from their eyes.
> In this world this edifice has been made;
> To display thereby the creator's glory.

No wonder Beau loved the Taj so much. This place is as powerful as Science and God. The Taj Mahal stands exactly as strong and perfect as it did in 1653. Nothing has atrophied in 335 years. My own brain can barely comprehend it. But this is what Asia taught my father and now me: *Believe in what cannot be fathomed.*

CHAPTER FOURTEEN

FORT ETHAN ALLEN

COLCHESTER, VERMONT

It is May 1998. I am thirty-three and married. My husband Allan Nicholls and I live in a condominium that used to be part of army officers' housing. Our building reminds me of my forefathers, which is unfortunate because I moved to Vermont to put some distance between me and Bercaws.

Ever since I returned from India, many years ago, I tested out life in a number of states—excluding Florida. After meeting Allan in Vermont, I decided to stay in Yankee Land with the Canadian man whom I married.

While we were courting, I took Allan to meet my father. I warned Al not to talk politics, past or present.

"Beau is very conservative," I said. "Don't tell him we are liberal Democrats."

"But that's not being true to yourself," Allan responded.

"I'm true to him."

Two years later finds me thinking of seceding from my union with Beau. I have received an invitation for his sixtieth birthday party and retirement celebration. Beau is leaving medicine. He doesn't like begging insurance companies for permission to order an MRI. He doesn't like the new trend of doctors bragging about how quickly they can see patients.

He is also increasingly worried about his own brain, although he's not articulating it. Beau has traded the *Journal of Neurology* in favor of *Life Extension* magazine.

"This is it, Gal. The fountain of youth. I've finally found it," he wrote in a recent letter.

Where do I fit in Beau's newly extended life? His sole focus is on his own brain.

I call Nora to tell her I can't make it down for the festivities.

"You're the only one who can't come," she says, sadly. "Kathy, Craig and Lee will be here."

"Nora, I don't think Beau even loves me anymore."

"What are you talking about? He calls you the child of his heart."

"Then why doesn't he ever ask me how I'm doing? Why doesn't he talk to me?"

Silence.

"Nora, all I do is listen to him—that is, of course, if he feels like saying anything. He's fine not uttering a word."

"Hang on a minute, Nan." Nora puts the phone down. I can hear her telling Beau to come to the kitchen. "*It's Nan,*" she whispers.

"Hi, Gal."

"Hi, Dad."

Silence. Nora whispers again: "*Ask her how she's doing.*"

"What?" Beau says into the receiver. "Hang on, Nancy, Nora's talking to me."

"*Beau, ask Nan how she is doing.*"

"Gal, Nora wants to know how you are doing."

"Tell Nora I'm fine but I can't make it to your party."

I hang up.

"This is not normal," I say to Allan after my botched phone call with Beau. "Parents are naturally interested in their children's lives. He couldn't care less."

"From what you've told me, he's never been normal, Nancy. This isn't a sudden, new development. This is who your father is. He doesn't like to talk, from what I can tell. And I can also tell that he loves you."

"Four years ago he asked me to shoot him if he turned out like his father. Guess what? He's him. It's official. I don't know if he actually has Alzheimer's or not, but he is becoming more remote like Berc did."

I should go to the goddamn party and poison his drink, which is what he swore me to do if he started acting like Berc. I want to be free of all this madness and obsession. But how? It's like trying not to have freckles when you're covered in them.

I boycott everything in Florida for the next few months. Craig's wedding. Nora's mother's funeral. I tell everyone, except Beau, that my father doesn't love me. No one knows what to say. No one ever knows what to say if it involves Dr. Beauregard Lee Bercaw.

A few months later, Allan and I are looking through an old photo album. There are a lot of pictures of Beau and me in Virginia.

"God, you look so much like your dad in this one," Allan says, pointing to one of us on a rock in the middle of the Rivanna. "Same legs, same kneecaps, same grin, same skin coloring...."

"Stop saying that!" I scream. "How can a woman look exactly like a man? I am nothing like him. I'd rather die than be like Beauregard."

"Nancy," Allan says, calmly. "You're saying the same thing he said about his father."

"Allan, do you know who Shah Jahan is?"

"Is he a rapper?" he laughs.

Allan makes films for a living. He's worked on almost every movie Robert Altman ever made. It occurs to me that he knows nothing about real life.

"Beau would call you a dumb-dumb," I lash out. "Shah Jahan built the Taj Mahal. He supposedly had this great love for his wife. Seems to me that he just loved the image of himself as a mogul. Shah Jahan means 'king of the world.' Beau thinks he's Shah Jahan, as well as the supreme Hindu god Vishnu. He had a sign on his office desk, next to his father's goddamn brain, which said, 'From the desk of God.'"

"Nancy, why don't you ever confront him? Fight back. Be true to you."

I did once, I explain to Allan, in high school. My boyfriend had gone to college. I told Beau and my mom that I was going to spend the night at my friend Wendy's house. Instead, I drove to Gainesville and had sex with Roger. I drove back the next morning and called Wendy from a payphone at a rest area to be sure everything was cool. She said that my dad was looking for me. I was in big trouble.

I arrived at home, and Beau was waiting for me. He was furious. He wanted to know where I had been. I told him that I had slept on the beach because I was depressed and needed time alone. He grilled me like I was on trial, as if he were a criminal lawyer: *What time did the sun rise? Did you have a sleeping bag? Where did you park?*

Unsatisfied with my vague responses, he sent my mother to get Wendy. He grilled her in front of me. He was rabid. Finally, I snapped. I looked right at him and said, "I hate you, Dad. When you come home, Lee and I hide. We'd rather not eat than see your face. You are the worst father in the world. I despise you."

"What did he do?" Allan asks.

"He looked perplexed at first. Like what I was saying couldn't possibly be true. Then, with the iciest stare I have ever seen, and in the most chilling tone I have ever heard, he said, 'I don't believe you.'"

"What happened then?"

"He stood up and left the room."

"Did you ever talk about it again?"

"Never. I found a condom in my father's lab coat a few days later and figured he was going to give it to me—that he knew what I had done. But a few days afterward we discovered he was having an affair with Nora. I think he'd attacked me because he was angry with his own deceit."

"Why did it take you twenty years to get mad at him?"

Tears are pouring down my face. "I guess I am afraid that one day soon I'll be the only Bercaw Filipino left. Alzheimer's disease is coming for Beau. I can hear it like a oncoming train. AD has a Doppler effect. He heard it. I hear it."

"What is it?" asks Allan, who played a heart surgeon in a film once.

"The pitch gets louder, more intense as it approaches. There's also something called a Doppler test, which uses ultrasonic waves to measure the blood's movement through veins. Any change in the wave means a blood clot might be present."

"How do you know this?'

"My dad taught me."

Allan tells me to call my dad and talk to him.

I dial Beau and Nora's number. Nora picks up, as usual.

"Hi, Nan! So nice to hear from you."

"Please put Beau on the phone."

"Beau," she yells, "it's your daughter!"

"Hi, ol' sweet Gal." He sounds weak.

"Dad, do you love me?"

"More than you'll ever know," he says, and sighs into the receiver.

"How was your party?"

"Here, I'll give the phone to Nora so she can tell you about it."

I sigh. Nora tells me how she filled the bathtub with champagne and everyone had a ball—especially Beau, who told stories from Kathmandu and Kenya.

"You should have heard how he talked about you, Nan. It sounded like you're a superhero or something."

CHAPTER FIFTEEN

DR. ANDERSON'S OFFICE

BURLINGTON, VERMONT

"Happy birthday to you. Happy birthday to you. Haaaaaappy bii-iiiirthday, sweet Gal. Your ol' dad sure loves you."

Beau calls me in Vermont first thing in the morning on my thirty-fourth birthday. It is December 27, 1998. He sings his variation of the song in his typical tone-deaf, non-rhyming way. But he doesn't hang up afterward. I am surprised that he keeps talking. I am used to dead air after his pronouncements.

"How does it feel to have lived half your life?"

"How does it feel to have a daughter this old?" I joke.

"I'm sending you a special present."

My father always sent great gifts. Even though my birthday was two days after Christmas, he never shortchanged me. In fact, he usually went overboard on both. On Christmas morning, when I was a kid, the living room was filled with presents from one end of the huge Oriental carpet to the other.

Some of the presents fulfilled my requests, like the time I got bouncy shoes with springs on them, but most fulfilled his idea of what I should have: light-up globes, atlases, the entire Nancy Drew collection, dictionaries, thesauri, encyclopedias, a subscription to *National Geographic*, a microscope and slides, binoculars, a telescope, a dinosaur-bone fossil set, the complete works of Shakespeare, the *Merck Manual* and a grow-your-own-brain-in-a-jar kit.

"What is it, Dad? I pretty much have everything I could possibly want."

"It's the genetic test for the Alzheimer's gene. It's very expensive. Take it to your doctor, have him draw the blood and return it to the genetic test company. But ask them to send the results to me."

"OK, thanks, Dad. I'm not sure I want to know, though," I laugh nervously. "I'd rather have diamonds, rubies and sapphires."

"You need to know, this is a gift of modern science. This is more important and valuable than jewelry," Beau barks at me.

"What if I have the genetic marker?" I ask.

"Start taking my supplement regimen and pray for a cure."

"Will you tell me the results?"

"Yes," he says.

"Allan is telling me that my breakfast is ready now. He's made me grits."

"Have a great birthday, Gal."

"Thanks for calling, Dad. I love you."

I can hear him sniff before hanging up the phone. I can tell he is worried about me. Will I go the way of Berc too? What had he wrought by bringing me into the world? A child with a death sentence?

He had the same tone upon handing me some paperwork to sign just before I boarded the plane for Kenya many years ago.

"What is this?" I had asked, knowing I shouldn't have.

"It's a one-million-dollar life-insurance policy," he said in a wobbly voice.

Even though he had raised me to be an adventurer, he knew the realities of malaria, bilharzias, and AIDS in Africa. After I signed it, he hugged me goodbye and walked away. Nora said he cried the whole way home, afraid he would actually get the money from his devil's bargain.

The test kit and a letter arrive a few days after our phone call, with a note.

Naples, Florida   January 4, 1999

Dear Gal,

   Re lab + ApoE, check all lab enclosed – fax to me + I'll tell you
what to do.
   I've corrected thru knowledge these problem – glycemic index,
IGF level, DHEA level as a result. Feel 10-15 years younger save
for prior damage – pray for me that I will be spared my father's +
brothers' affliction + that I will be able to go back to work to uti-
lize all this knowledge.

                        Much love,
                        Dad

   His brothers' affliction, too? I guess Beau believes none of them is
exempt from Berc's legacy.
   I take the instructions and test kit to my physician, Dr. Anderson,
who draws my blood and ships it off. Dr. Anderson seems happy
enough to comply with my father's wishes. But he also recommends
the name of a good psychiatrist.
   I send my father a thank you note for the test kit. Thank you letters
were vitally important to Beau. One must show gratitude for gifts
and kindness. I wasn't allowed to play with any gifts from Christmas
or my birthday until the letters were written and in the mail to everyone who had sent one.
   The letters couldn't just say, *"Thank you for the _____. I love it. I
hope you had a nice Christmas. I miss you. Love, Nan."* They had to
be full of news and take up the entire space inside the note card and
be written in my best cursive. My Christmas stocking always held
the season's supply of holiday-themed thank you cards—no excuse
to wait.
   It takes me a long time to come up with the right way to thank
Beau for the genetic test. A test I didn't want in the first place, but
felt helpless to protest against. Beau was dead set on me getting it.

Dear Dad,

This is a very thought-provoking gift. The gift of knowing whether or not I might forget. I don't know what to say. The other day I was recalling our safari in Kenya and how much fun that was. I hope to go back to Africa some day and see how it's changed. But I'd also like to see the temples of Angkor Wat in Cambodia. What's your favorite place on earth? Another great gift would be for us to go there together. I vote for the Amazon. We could hire a captain and go the length. One of those encyclopedias you gave me says that the Amazon is longer than the Nile. I bet we would see anaconda and crocodile. Personally, I wouldn't want to swim in the Amazon, considering the piranhas and the crazy bacteria—or is it small fish?—that swim up your urethra and kill you. I'll look it up and get back to you. My guess is that you would like to see the Philippines again. Come to think of it, so would I.

Love, Gal

P.S. I looked it up. It's a tiny parasitic catfish that swims up a urine stream and lodges in the urethra by expanding its barbs. The Amazon is out. The Philippines are in.

I want to ask my father if he had given my brother the same test kit. But I already know the answer is no. Lee is not Beau's clone. The Rixey blood had diluted his physical resemblance to us, thus suggesting his ApoE DNA had been tempered as well.

Dr. No would inherit the Rixey receding hairline and high blood pressure. My father and I would lose our minds in the vicinity of our own heads. We were linked like Chang and Eng, the famous Siamese twins who shared a piece of cartilage at their sternum. I imagined that my father and I were conjoined by the neural fibers connecting the two hemispheres of the brain. We were of one mind in the way Chang and Eng were of one body.

Before my father could have even received my thank you letter, I get the call. I am in the middle of coaching swim practice at the University of Vermont when someone comes down from the athletic director's office to say that my father needed to speak with me urgently. How had he found the number?

"Hi, Dad."

"Hi, Gal, bad news."

"What?"

"Your test shows that you are the same as me."

"I think we expected that," I say. "What does the test say?"

"We both carry ApoE 3."

"What does that mean exactly?"

"It means we may or may not get the disease."

"That's good news," I say.

"No, it's not."

"Dad, I have to get back to the team."

Beau and I were no better off knowing our test results than not knowing. Regardless, my father interpreted the outcome as: *You will get what I get, and I will get what my father got.* Yet, somehow, I didn't care. I swore to myself that Beau's obsession would not become mine—even if I am destined for Alzheimer's too.

CHAPTER SIXTEEN

LYLES BAPTIST CHURCH

PALMYRA, VIRGINIA

The year is 2002; I am thirty-six. My grandmother, who is ninety-seven, is dying in her apartment at Our Lady of Peace Nursing Home in Charlottesville. Beau has crossed out her nurse's food orders and prescribed his own protocol.

"Key lime pie only." Her favorite, and the only kind she couldn't make to perfection.

Four years earlier, in 1998, Grandmother sold Rebelanna. Her eldest son, Woodson, was outraged. He was meant to inherit the property.

But something—or someone—caused Grandmother to change her mind. Beau supported her decision, as did his brother David. Woodson and Peter were furious. The sale of Rebelanna launched a Civil War between Bercaw brothers.

When the new owners arrived at the farm with their moving trucks, Woodson was waiting for them. He was standing on the front lawn with a rifle. The police were called, but the new owners didn't press charges.

Grandmother had raised her four wild sons without much help from her husband. Berc was either at war, in Washington, or succumbing to Alzheimer's. When he was home, and before he lost his mind, he was a tyrant. He would beat the boys, and Grandmother, just to remind them who was in charge. The farm had been their refuge. They could play with Berc when he was in a good state of mind and they could run from him when he wasn't. My father stated his affection for the farm in many letters to his mother.

University of Florida, Gainesville   10 December 1967

Dear Nancy,

Hope everything is going OK with Berc. I don't know exactly why, but I agree it would be wise to keep the farm—sure do like the farm. But do whatever is best for you. Also hope that you don't try to keep Berc longer than you're able. Dr. Johns said to me that you appeared to be under a big strain + was concerned about your health.

Love,
Beau + Barbara

At the end of Grandmother's life, the Bercaw sons—except for David, who passed away suddenly from septicemia shortly after the farm was sold—were causing her troubles all over again. Woodson wanted his share of her money—a small fortune amassed entirely from Ralston Purina stock—before she died, so that he could pay for a new house since the farm was gone. Peter wanted whatever Woodson wanted, and Beau wanted the opposite of whatever his brothers did. Grandmother, non-confrontational by nature, was trapped in the middle. She tended to agree with whomever she spoke with last.

Three years before her 100th birthday, Grandmother decided it was time to end all the conflict. She told the nurses that her death was imminent. They, in turn, told the brothers. Each morning, from the time of her announcement to the time of her death, Grandmother got up and put on her makeup and finest clothes. She sat in an arm chair and waited all day for people to come pay their respects. Beau was there by the second day, serving her Key lime pie, even though she refused to eat.

I arrived from Vermont on the fifth day. Cousin Nancy had already been there, as had Uncle Woodson and Uncle Pete, and just about everyone with the last name Bercaw or who lived in Palmyra.

Grandmother said hardly a word to me when it was my turn. I just sat next to her and held her hand. She looked regal in a bright blue suit jacket and skirt. She wore her pearls and blue hat. She even wore stockings. I was grief stricken when I left her room, knowing that I would never see her alive again. I had spent nearly every summer of my life with her, and some winters too, when she would come down to Florida to escape the snow.

To me, she will always be sitting in the kitchen at the farm, before sunrise, sipping coffee and smoking one cigarette (she had another at night) while the pie she made for breakfast baked. I used to get up early on vacation just to see her like that and spend time alone with her. She would listen to music, or the local news, and lean back in her wicker chair and whistle along to whatever song was on. Once in a great while, she would lean back too far in the chair and fall over. But she had lived her life on the precipice between her violent husband and her hellion sons. Perhaps she was at home there.

No matter what happened to her, though, Grandmother never complained. Even if the pipes were frozen, or she had pneumonia, or the furnace broke. She just went about her business. When a bear ran across the front yard once, Grandmother got the shotgun off the wall and took aim. She missed the bear and then returned to her coffee and radio. As she told me the story, I was sure she missed on purpose. Grandmother was too gentle. She called her housekeeper "my good Eleanor," and when Eleanor was too old to work, Grandmother gave her a pension.

Whenever I whined about a skinned knee or a breakup with a boyfriend, Grandmother had one thing to say: *Poor, pitiful little thing.* I knew she was being comforting and chiding at the same time—a Bercaw specialty, even though technically she wasn't a Bercaw, except by marriage. She was a Scott who raised Bercaws.

Beau, the physician, was with her at the end. I had gone back home to Vermont, only to get the call a few days later. My father could barely speak.

"Your grandmother has gone to heaven," was all he said on the phone, as if I were eleven and not thirty-six.

Nora called back later to tell me that funeral arrangements were being made. Grandmother would be buried at Lyles Baptist Church between her husband and son David. She wanted a simple head-stone that simply stated her name, as well as her birth and death dates.

Nora went on to say that, in his grief, Beau was insisting on a gi-gantic granite tombstone that contained every word of the Prayer of St. Francis of Assisi in huge letters.

Lord, make me an instrument of your peace.
Where there is hatred, let me sow love.
Where there is injury, pardon.
Where there is doubt, faith.
Where there is despair, hope.
Where there is darkness, light.
Where there is sadness, joy.
O Divine Master,
grant that I may not so much seek to be consoled, as to console;
to be understood, as to understand;
to be loved, as to love.
For it is in giving that we receive.
It is in pardoning that we are pardoned,
and it is in dying that we are born to Eternal Life.

Fortunately, Nora kept reminding Beau of Grandmother's wishes for a simple grave marker—a big one would overwhelm Lyles' tiny graveyard. Finally, he capitulated. I was surprised. Beau never gave up once he got an idea in his head.

Lyles Baptist Church is filled when I walk in with Allan. My father is in the front row with Nora. Woodson is there with his new wife

Karen. Brother Pete is beside them. My cousin Nancy and her two brothers are in the row in front of me, next to David's widow Penny and daughter Kathy along with her young daughters. Allan and I sit with Aunt Sue, Woodson's ex-wife. Every seat in the church is filled.

The minister says a few words about Grandmother before introducing my father, who reads a psalm per Grandmother's request. We sing one of Grandmother's favorite hymns and then Woodson takes the podium. The program states that he will be reading a poem by Tennyson. The entire service was planned by Grandmother long before her death.

"Instead of the poem listed," Woodson begins, "I'd like to read a poem that I wrote for my grandmother, Nannie Dunlap Scott."

Woodson doesn't get very far into his poem before launching into another tangent.

"My mother should have been more like her mother. Nancy was not a good mother. She should have punished us more. She let us get away with too much. I blame her for my problems. My brother David was the worst. She didn't discipline him when Berc was away."

Cousin Nancy puts her arm around cousin Kathy. Woodson is condemning Kathy's dead father, as well as his own dead mother, at her funeral.

I see Beau put his head in his hands.

I look at Allan. He looks back in disbelief.

Woodson, in full military uniform with all his medals on his chest, is now pacing back and forth in front of the altar. He is working himself into frenzy. He keeps referring to some notes.

"I still can't believe my own mother sold the farm out from under me. And those people who bought it! I offered to pay them $50,000 more than they paid to get it back. They refused. What kind of selfish, horrible people are they? I can't believe I fought in two wars to protect this country and people like them."

Those people are in attendance. The Barbers get up and leave. Woodson is emboldened by the victory. His voice rises and his pace increases. He rambles on and on. I go numb.

"What kind of person takes her eldest son's home and birthright away?" He continues. "What kind of...."

Cousin Nan tries to interrupt him.

"Father. Father. Father. Father. Father. Father. Father. Father."

Finally, he looks at her.

"This is about Grandmother," Nan says.

"I'm talking about her," he barks, angrily awakened from a diatribe-induced trance.

The minister, who once lived with his wife in the tiny guesthouse on the Bercaw farm, seizes the moment to put his arm around Woodson and move the funeral along. I stare at my own father. I can't believe he has done nothing. He just sits there brain-dead while Woodson curses their mother. I don't know who is more infuriating.

The minister asks if anyone would like to say something about Nancy Scott Bercaw. One man stands up and tells the crowd how he had never known a more loving soul.

"Mrs. Bercaw noticed a kid in Sunday School who had a club foot. She spoke to his parents, who couldn't afford to have it fixed. Mrs. Bercaw drove that boy into Charlottesville for doctor's appointments and surgery, and paid for it all out of her own pocket. That little boy was me."

I am hysterical. I don't understand what is real. Was my grandmother a sinner or a saint? This is what Bercaws do: muddy the waters until you can't see what you are swimming in—and you drown from panic.

When the service ends, I run outside to find cousin Nan. She is smoking and crying under a tree behind the church. I grab the cigarette from her lips and inhale. It's like we are little girls all over again: stealing Grandmother's cigarettes when everyone else is asleep. Grandmother knew, of course, but never said a thing about it. She just filled up her cigarette holder all over again.

"There's only one thing to say," I tell my favorite cousin, the other Nancy Bercaw. "This makes it official. The Bercaws are crazier than the Bells. Crazier than any character Faulkner could have written. Let's be proud of that, shall we?"

She lets out a good long laugh. The Bells lived in Palmyra too, in a dilapidated house that they let their cows walk through. Grandmother used to pay their taxes so that they wouldn't lose their home.

Nan and I go back to the church basement where Grandmother's friends from around Fluvanna County have set out a lunch. Except for the bustling of china and some whispering, it is very quiet. I fill up my plate with ham, cabbage and cornbread—all the food Grandmother used to make for me. I sit down with Kent and Harriet Loving. They have been my grandmother's friends and accountants for forty years. Kent's mother lived in the same nursing home in Charlottesville.

Harriet looks at me mournfully and shakes her head.

Woodson walks in and goes right to the buffet line. The minister breaks the silence with a prayer. My father and Nora leave immediately afterward.

Later that afternoon, Allan and I have an early dinner with Beau and Nora at Grandmother's favorite restaurant, the Village Inn, near the famed Fort Union Military Academy for wayward boys. My father utters one statement before his fried catfish is served.

"I will never speak to Woodson again in my life."

Allan and I go to Woodson's house after dinner. Woodson is parked in front of the television, watching *Law and Order,* sipping his umpteenth Maker's Mark on the rocks and chain-smoking Salem menthol cigarettes.

Cousin Nan is in the backyard doing pretty much the same thing, without the TV. I join her.

Nancy tells me that she had been to lunch with her father and brothers, as well as her mother *and* Karen, after the ceremony.

"What happened?"

"Father asked us if we thought what he did was right."

"What did you say?"

"Nobody said anything. He launched into a new discourse on why he was right."

"Who's gonna write about this, cuz?" I ask. Nancy is a professor of Southern American history at Ole Miss. I am a journalist now. I can feel this thing between our fathers getting between us. I don't want it to happen.

"Probably you," she says.

"Maybe we should write it together. The Nancy Bercaws. What it's like growing up with Woodson and Beauregard as our fathers, and being named for their mother."

Nancy cuts me off. "She shouldn't have sold the farm."

"I know."

"She didn't need the money to pay for Our Lady of Peace."

"I know." Grandmother had come to Florida once with $30,000 cash in her purse just in case she wanted to buy a new car.

"Now none of us has the farm."

Beau had encouraged Grandmother to sell the farm for one reason only: he didn't want Woodson to have it.

"He'll ruin it," Beau told me once. "We should sell it to someone who will take care of it."

I had agreed, like I always did.

The day after the funeral, my father calls the Barbers to ask if we can go swimming in the Rivanna River. Even though Woodson had upset them, they loved Beau—who had sent them a long letter telling them the history of the farm. He had also sent me a copy of the letter, so I would remember too.

Dear Mr. and Mrs. Barber,

Eight days ago, my wife, Nora, and I flew into Charlottesville to see my ailing mother, Nancy Bercaw, and to say goodbye to the farm, which we had named Rebelanna. The river that runs through it is called Rivanna, named for the Queen Anne. With my father and mother being from the south, they named the farm

Rebelanna, in part after their heritage and part after the river and Queen Anne. As our flight lowered over the Rivanna River, tears came to my eyes, as the river and the farm will always be a treasure in my life.

I write to you for two major reasons. The first is to apologize for what I have heard were inappropriate (and probably worse) actions and deeds of my eldest brother, Woodson. He certainly does not speak for the rest of the family, and I believe he has embarrassed even his closest friends in Fluvanna County.

Second and more important I want to welcome you to Rebelanna (or whatever name you wish to call it) and to tell you about the farm and the folks that were there—both past and present.

First and foremost, my mother, Nancy Dunlap Scott Bercaw, lived there from 1941 to 1996 or 1997 when she moved to an ACLF in Charlottesville. Nana (which I affectionately call her now) is a living example of St. Francis' prayer; that is, able to turn aside venom with love and concern. I have witnessed her do this a number of times with her family and others and, most recently, with her eldest son Woodson. She has been and always shall be the inspiration of my life.

The Rivanna River: Down the hill is one of the world's greatest swimming holes. It has grown up now with poison ivy and needs to be cleared. We had a rope that hung from a tree and hung over the river so we could drop like Tarzan into the water. The large rock to the right of the swimming hole was called "snake rock" for obvious reasons, a problem that could be easily solved by boys with .22 rifles. I used to swim with snakes in the river and 99/100 were no problems.

The hardest thing I ever did in my life was being required by my folks to drown our kittens. The cat population was getting out of control. Scrawny sadly later died from what was the rat control program by my father, using Coumadin. Coumadin not only killed the rats, but my cat and also was used as therapy on my Aunt Louise and was the cause of her death as well. I am happy to say that even though it was recommended for my mother because of her heart condition, I opposed it. I did not want everyone in my family to die from it. I know for a fact that it has already saved her life twice by the fact of not being on it.

Why am I telling you all of this? Rebelanna desperately needs someone to love it and to care for it. Otherwise, it will too be reclaimed by the wilderness, as have all the other places. Everything that I have heard about you is good, and I hope that you will enjoy and love the farm as much as we did. Neither I or any of my brothers are able to give it the required care now. Therefore, I am happy for someone like you to have it, even though we are all, especially me, emotionally attached to the place.

Sincerely,
Beau Bercaw

I call cousin Nan and tell her to come to Rebelanna. She brings her brothers. Together, we splash around and laugh like kids. Beau does too.

A few weeks later, Beau calls me at my house in Vermont.

"Remember, Gal, if I wind up like my brothers, shoot me. You promised."

He *was* acting like his brothers. I don't answer him. He isn't listening anyway. I hang up. I had promised Beau that I would kill him *only* if he wound up like his father. I should just take out a .22 rifle and aim for everyone with my same last name. Instead, I decide to move to Virginia and, once there, try to add another Bercaw to the family.

III

The Ending

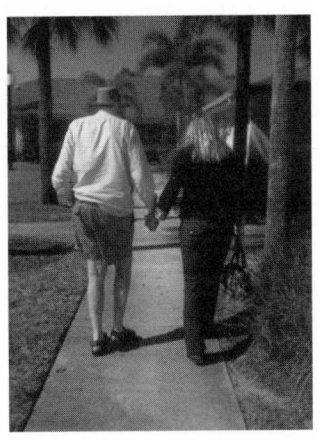

*In examining disease, we gain wisdom
about anatomy and physiology and biology.
In examining the person with disease,
we gain wisdom about life.*

—Oliver Sacks, MD

CHAPTER SEVENTEEN

ROCKINGHAM MEMORIAL HOSPITAL

HARRISONBURG, VIRGINIA

I look out the window of the delivery room at 3 p.m. on March 21, 2004. I am thirty-eight and I finally agreed to an epidural after eighteen hours of labor.

"Look, Allan, snow! In Virginia! In March!" I say, before throwing up in one of those stupid pink kidney-shaped pans.

"Nancy, it's time to push," my Filipino doctor says. She is an old-fashioned doctor, the kind who delivers babies and then becomes their pediatrician. Like a veterinarian. How did she get to Harrisonburg, Virginia, from Manila? Allan and I had moved here so I could be the head coach of women's swimming at James Madison University, my mother's alma mater. I happened to call the lone obstetrician in Rockingham County who was originally from the Philippines.

When my grandmother died, I decided that someone named Nancy Bercaw must always live in Virginia. Cousin Nancy was happily ensconced in Oxford, Mississippi, so I took my own mandate to heart. My dad was thrilled to hear I was moving to the Shenandoah Valley. He told me how he and his University of Virginia pals, John Eagle and Al Justice, used to drive from Charlottesville to Harrisonburg on the weekends to meet girls at JMU.

Dr. Nio asks me to push again.

"How can I push if I can't feel the lower half of my body?"

I like thinking of my child swimming around in amniotic fluid, resisting life on dry land. A little mermaid reluctant to trade in her tailfin for a life of suffering.

"Imagine that you can," Dr. Nio says.

I push, and count, and push again.

"Good, Nancy."

Dr. Nio is manipulating my baby's head through the birth canal. I hope my baby isn't stuck. This is how children are born with cerebral palsy.

"Again," she says. "Push."

"Are you a neurologist?" I ask her. "We may need one if this baby goes without oxygen for any period of time."

"Push," she says calmly.

"You remind me of my father," I tell her.

"Come on, Nancy, a few more pushes."

I comply.

"It's a boy!" she says.

Allan cuts the cord. While the nurses are cleaning up our baby, I stare at the boy's tiny face. His eyes are puffy. I wonder if he has Down syndrome.

I ask Dr. Nio if my baby is healthy.

"Perfectly."

"He doesn't have an extra copy of chromosome 21?"

Dr. Nio is too busy sewing me up to answer. Maybe I hadn't even said it out loud.

"Nancy," Allan says, well aware of what I am thinking or saying. "His eyes are puffy because he's a Bercaw. He looks just like you."

"What are we gonna name him?" I ask.

Allan and I had picked two girl names: Fiona or Virginia. Allan has two boys from his previous marriage: John and Andrew. Both live back in Vermont with their mother.

"I'd like to call him David after my brother," Allan says. His brother had died many years earlier, like my Uncle David.

"David Beauregard Nicholls," I announce before falling asleep. "That's his name."

My mother is in the waiting room. She came from Florida for the birth, timing her arrival perfectly. I imagined this was a strange day for Barbara. Thirty-eight years earlier, while she was giving birth to me at Clark Air Base, her mother was dying in Culpeper, Virginia— about sixty miles from where we are now.

Allan calls Beau and Nora.

"We had a baby boy this afternoon," he tells Nora. "Nancy wanted me to tell you that he is a true Southern gentleman, born at 5 p.m. on a Sunday. Suppertime. He's long and lean, just like a Bercaw. His name is David Beauregard."

Nora relays the information to Beau, who is doing Sudoku in his big leather chair. She shares Beau's response with Allan.

"He got the sweetest look on his face, and a tear fell down his cheek," Nora says, choking up herself. "We'll drive up next week."

As soon as I am released, my mother helps us get David Beau home and settled. She makes us meals and rubs my back. I have a pit in my stomach about my baby. How am I going to keep him alive and well? I don't know how to breathe, let alone function. Will this feeling last my whole life?

When Barbara goes back to Florida, Beau and Nora drive up.

Beau walks into my house sheepishly. When he sees me holding David, his eyes get big. I hand him my baby.

"Hold your grandson," I say. "Your namesake. Talk to him."

Beau cradles David close to his face. In a cooing voice, he says, "Your ol' granddad sure loves you."

Two days later, we go to Lyles Baptist Church in Palmyra. I have arranged to have David Beauregard blessed where his ancestors were buried: Grandmother Nancy, Grandfather Berc and Uncle David. I want to overwrite the last time we were here, when Uncle Woodson lost his mind during a eulogy to his mother.

The new minister is excited to meet the infamous Bercaws. A dozen or so of Grandmother's old friends come too, including Harriett and Kent Loving, who are still managing the remains of her estate.

At my request, Beau reads a scripture of his choosing. He selects Mark 10:10-13 to honor the occasion. I listen intently.

> And in the house his disciples asked him again of the same matter. And he saith unto them, Whosoever shall put away his wife, and marry another, committeth adultery against her. And if a woman shall put away her husband, and be married to another, she committeth adultery.

I look at Allan. It's happening again—another Bercaw is going insane at Lyles Baptist Church in front of everyone. Beau is reading a passage about adultery. Thankfully, he continues and the next passage is appropriate.

> And they brought young children to him, that he should touch them: and his disciples rebuked those that brought them. But when Jesus saw it, he was much displeased, and said unto them, Suffer the little children to come unto me, and forbid them not: for of such is the kingdom of God. Verily I say unto you, Whosoever shall not receive the kingdom of God as a little child, he shall not enter therein. And he took them up in his arms, put his hands upon them, and blessed them.

After the ceremony, the people who own the old farm, the Barbers, invite us over for a champagne toast.

"Look at Rebelanna!" I exclaim as we drive up the gravel driveway. The lawn is lush green and perfectly groomed. Two horses stand in the front field. The house has a fresh coat of white paint. It shimmers in the afternoon sun.

"It's like the Taj Mahal," mutters Beau, who is sitting next to me.

I notice that he has a wet spot on his pants. I am not sure whether he has noticed or not. When we get out of the car, Nora helps him to the bathroom "to freshen up."

A few minutes later they join us on the back porch, where we all look out at the Rivanna River. The Barbers have cut down trees and cleared the fields to have an unobstructed view. I am torn between the sight of the river and the sight of my father staring longingly at it.

I can feel Beau remembering his canoe and his shotgun. I can feel his legs jumping off the rocks in the deep swimming hole. I can feel his arms hold onto the rope swing and letting go. And I can feel my father slipping away from me, just as the farm slipped away from us.

CHAPTER EIGHTEEN

FIRST METHODIST CHURCH

NAPLES, FLORIDA

It is March 30, 2006, and I have just returned from getting my son's first haircut. He is two and I am forty-one. We had moved back to Vermont from Virginia a few months after he was born. We wanted to be near Allan's older sons, so we could be one big family.

After I put David down for a nap, I notice a blinking light on the answering machine. I push play.

"Gal, is that you? Gal? Um, are you there? Call your father. Call Beau. Call me."

Answering machines confuse my dad. As many times as we have explained it to him, he couldn't tell the difference between a real voice and a taped version. I think he didn't much care one way or another. What was odd is that he called. Usually Nora does that for him.

I call Beau back, excited to tell him about David's first haircut. My son looks more like a Bercaw than ever. Beau will get a big kick out of that.

"Hi, Dad, it's Gal!" I say excitedly.

"Craig is dead."

"What?" He can't mean my stepbrother.

"Craig put a shotgun to his head and pulled the trigger this morning."

"Where is Nora?"

"She's here with our minister."

"Dad, I'll call you back later. I need to hang up now."

The world is spinning. I lie on my stomach on the floor afraid I might rotate off into space.

I crawl downstairs to my computer, where an email from stepsister Kathy is waiting for me. The subject line reads: 911. There is no message in the body when I open it.

I Google "*Craig Richard Marshall, Collier County Sheriff's Department.*"

News of his suicide, and rapid fall from police-force grace, is all over the Naples news' outlets. Television reporters are in front of his house. The sheriff is saying, "I did everything I could for that boy."

I had only recently discovered that Craig had a serious drug addiction. He had been to rehab twice in the past year—a fact that came to my attention only through a strange series of events that also made the headlines.

Four weeks earlier, Craig had been on routine police duty when he was shot in the back of his shoulder. He called the crime in to his station, which then put all schools in Craig's proximity on lockdown. A manhunt ensued.

Craig's wound was superficial and he was discharged from the hospital after getting bandaged up. He was a hero—until the sheriff's office pieced the story together twenty-four hours later. The wound had come from Craig's own gun. But why did he do it, and why did he lie? Moreover, how had he managed to shoot himself from behind?

Craig came clean with Nora, saying that he was sick of his desire for drugs, which was potent in the minutes before he pulled the trigger. By replacing the craving with pain, he had hoped to conquer it. But after shooting his shoulder, Craig panicked—radioing in that a sniper had hit him. Shot in the line of duty, he hoped to play it, rather than out of desperation.

Nora and Beau admitted Craig into the psychiatric ward of Naples

Community Hospital to rescue him from withdrawal, as well as the sheriff's wrath.

Craig went back to work after a few days in the hospital despite the fact that he was under investigation for fraud. Craig told Nora he was ready to accept responsibility, and whatever the consequences, he would face them. Everything was going to change. He had learned his lesson, lots of lessons. No more drugs; no more lies.

Two weeks later, Craig is dead. And I am staring at a computer screen full of news about him. I call Kathy.

"It's Nan," I say through a tidal wave of sorrow. "I know. Beau told me. I got his message before I saw your email. I'm reading the coverage. I love you. I am so sorry, Kathy. What happened?"

"He got arrested for a DUI two nights ago. They locked him up and then let him go in the morning. The sheriff fired him on the spot."

"Then what?"

"This morning he called Mom and asked her to help him get his truck out of impound. After he hung up, he taped paper to the windows. Then, well, you know what he did."

"That's what Nora walked into when she got there?"

Kathy can't speak anymore. She had been calling family all morning, in her best matter-of-fact voice—a ruse she can no longer maintain.

"Where are you?" I asked. She lives in North Carolina with her husband and daughters.

"I'm in Florida with the girls and Paul. I came here to check on Craig. I was so worried. He wasn't returning my calls. I was afraid this might happen. But he did it before I could get to him. We're at a hotel in Naples."

"I'll be there soon," I tell her and hang up.

I call Lee, who is a cop in Tampa.

"What have you heard about Craig?" I ask.

"It's a mess," he said. "A nightmare."

"How is Beau going to help Nora through this?" I ask my brother.

"He's no stranger to death."

"Clinically speaking."

"He'll handle it like he did his mother's death."

"By saying nothing? That won't help Nora."

"Just being there is enough. There's nothing anyone can say or do to make it better anyway."

"Lee, I don't know if you're paying attention or not, but Beau isn't the man he was when we were kids. He's not Gator Man anymore. All he does is math. He's so afraid of Alzheimer's that he doesn't actually engage with humans anymore. Maybe he's even in the early stages and no one is talking about it."

"Nancy, Craig is dead. Don't make this about Beau."

"I'm not. I'm trying to figure out how to help Nora in light of our father's shortcomings."

"You can't."

"What are the Tampa cops saying about Craig?"

"We've seen this before, sadly. Profound drug addiction is almost incurable. Beau told us that."

Indeed, Beau had taken great pains to warn us kids, in a long handwritten letter, about the dangers of unsafe sex and drug abuse, complete with medical literature on AIDS and addiction. I got the original during my first year in college. Beau photocopied the letter for Lee, Kathy and Craig, who were all in high school at the time — just as Berc had once used carbon paper when he typed so that he could send the same letter to all of his sons whenever communicating difficult information.

Interestingly, Beau had never warned us about guns. Yet he had cautioned Grandmother about them in a letter about Berc's declining condition.

> Don't let Emily or anyone else sway you about moving away from the farm with Berc. I think you know by sad experience how he reacts to strange uncertain conditions. This is characteristic of the disease. The farm is surely the best place for him until you can

manage him no longer. Concerning Mrs. Brooks's fears, I think it probably would be a very good idea to remove the guns in the house or have them made inoperable....

Berc wasn't allowed to accidentally shoot himself, but Beau made me swear to put a gun to his head if he turned out like his father. Now, all of a sudden, my sweet stepbrother is dead by a self-inflicted gunshot to his head. I am so mixed up, and so desperately want to assign blame.

I ask my brother when he learned that Craig had a drug problem.

"Only recently."

"Same here."

"Clearly, it's not just Beau who has trouble talking about things," Lee says.

"Yes, brother, it's all of us," I say. "I'll get to Florida as soon as I can. Call me if there is anything I should know, OK? No more silence on this or any subject."

I hear David singing in his crib and walk upstairs.

Before your nap, baby Beau, the world was one way. Now it's another. You will never know your Uncle Craig. The ten-year-old boy I met in a van on the way to Virginia early one morning twenty-four years ago is gone.

Beau had taught Craig and Lee, as well as me and Kathy, how to fire guns on the farm that first summer. Three years later, the boys got into big trouble for shooting out all the windows on the old cars in the barn. Ten years later, they both became cops.

I arrive in Naples two days later in anticipation of Craig's memorial service. Kathy picks me up at the airport and tries to fill me in on what's happening and how everyone is dealing with it. She is tired and weepy. I am scared to see Nora. I ask Kathy what to expect.

"Mom is very shaky. She keeps talking about how she found Craig. She called the minister immediately, who happened to be at the church. Then she called the police. She was there when the sheriff came."

"Then, what happened?"

"The sheriff was defensive. Claimed he'd done all he could for Craig."

Tears are getting caught in my throat. I can't imagine Nora having to deal with the sheriff's bullshit on top of her son's death. It's too much. I pray Beau is being helpful in some way—and is not immersed in puzzles and math. Nora needs him to listen, or at the very least, be present.

"So," Kathy continues, "because Craig technically wasn't a cop at the time of his death, the sheriff is threatening not to let the department's Bugle Corps play 'Taps' at his funeral. He's refusing to give Craig that one final act of respect. It's a fucking disaster."

Kathy is planning the service with Craig's ex-wife, Leslie, who had divorced him because of the drugs although she still loved him. We pull into the driveway, where Nora's sister Trish greets us. Kathy is trying very hard to hold herself together. I admire her ability to function in a time of crisis. I feel like I might fall to my knees at any moment and never get up again.

"Nancy, great to see you," Trish says.

I don't know what to say back to her. All words seem useless. Trish is married to my father's former colleague, Dr. Weems Hollowell— a neurosurgeon who is still operating on brains and spinal cords.

Before Weems married Trish, and before Beau married Nora, Weems's daughter drowned in his backyard pool, just a few houses down from us. Weems and Beau raced back from the office when the news came in, along with every other doctor who lived on Harbor View Lane. They tried what the paramedics had attempted in vain. Afterward, Beau ran over to our house and called me down from the tree house. He pulled me into his giant embrace.

"Lynn Hollowell is dead. She broke her spine diving into a shallow pool," he cried in agony. "Promise me you won't ever do that, Gal. Promise me. Always go feet first into water. Swear to me, Gal. Swear."

Beau fell back in the grass and screamed bloody murder. Lynn was four years older than me. Her sixteenth birthday had been a week away. Many years later, we learned that Lynn's death might have been suicide.

Now Craig was dead too, before his thirty-fifth year.

"Where's Nora?" I ask Trish.

"She's getting her nails done. Her manicurist came over to do them for her. I was just going to get some veggie platters at Publix."

I don't know how anyone has the strength to function.

"Where's my dad?" I ask.

"He's in his chair."

I go upstairs into Nora and Beau's condo—now a mausoleum of the lives that used to be here: framed pictures of cheetahs on the Serengeti at dusk, the Taj Mahal at sunrise, the Great Pyramid at Giza in the noon-day sun, and the spear given to my father by the Maragoli tribe.

I stop to look at the piano. There is a picture of Craig smiling on his honeymoon, a can of Bud Light in his hand and a fishing pole dipping into the Gulf of Mexico behind him.

Beau is in his recliner doing math. He stands up when he sees me.

"Hi, Gal." His voice is sad. He puts one arm around me.

"Where's Nora?" I ask, bursting into tears. "Are you helping her?"

My father looks puzzled by the second question, and points to the porch.

Nora is getting her nails done. I try to hug her while she stays seated. I try not to mess up the polish. She is weepy and in another world. She looks at me, confused.

"Nora, I love you. We'll get through this. I'll wait for you inside."

She nods tearfully.

I wonder if Dad has given her something, or if grief has shut her down. There are enough prescription drugs in this house to turn Naples into Jonestown. I had taken advantage of that fact a number of times in my own life. Beau had a great drug to treat tension headaches, which I discovered could erase a hangover in five minutes. One day I read the warning label, which said that "organic brain disease" was a potential side effect, and I never took another one.

Kathy is at the computer researching a song for the service.

"I don't understand anything any more," I tell her. "I feel like this is the beginning of the end for all of us. Our family used to be quirky, but now we're ruined."

"Yup," she says, nodding her head.

The doorbell rings. It's the minister, come to check on us.

I escort him past the pictures of the lives formerly known as ours, to the couch in the living room. Beau turns into a Southern gentleman for our guest. "We sure appreciate you coming by," he says.

Nora comes in from the porch and the nail lady leaves. Trish is back with the veggie platters, and is rearranging boxes of wine in the refrigerator to make room for them. We all gather in the living room, as the minister instructs, and hold hands.

I close my eyes as he begins a prayer for us.

"Please help the Bercaws in this time of crisis. Give them the strength and courage to help each other. Let them know that Craig is safe in your arms now...."

At the funeral the next morning, Lee sits next to me. Nora and Beau are in front of us with their former daughter-in-law Leslie. Kathy is on the other side of her mother with her kids and husband. Craig's father and stepmother are with us too.

A man sings "On Wings of Eagles," the song Kathy picked out.

Pictures of Craig line the altar: fishing in the Everglades; at Kathy's wedding in Newport; with his grandmother somewhere; and in a canoe with me at my grandmother's farm. There is no coffin because Craig was cremated—along with his cowboy boots.

Kathy has found a company that blends ashes with concrete to create living reefs for the bottom of the ocean. She has ordered a plaque for Craig's that says "Gone Fishing." Eventually we will take his "reef ball," as they are named, out to sea.

Meanwhile, the church is a sea of police-uniform blue. My brother, in his uniform, looks as cold and sweaty as the string beans he eschewed some twenty-five years ago—before Craig came into our lives and charmed us all with his quirky *joie de vivre*.

Seems like minutes ago we were in the Rivanna River: Beau warning us about cottonmouths, tipping the canoe, and eating Snickers.

Craig had moved up through the ranks of the force—from prison guard to police officer—and Beau was mighty proud of him. Craig was his "good ol' boy."

Someone says a prayer.

> God our refuge and strength,
> close at hand in our distress;
> meet us in our sorrow and lift our eyes
> to the peace and light of your constant care.

People take turns saying things about Craig.

"He was a good friend."

"He was a kind person."

"He had a heart of gold."

Beau says nothing and I feel like I have to overcompensate for him. I get up and talk about the honor of calling Craig my brother and I tell everyone how he once saved the life of a choking infant. I tell people about our fun times canoeing in Virginia. I say it as much for my father's ears as everyone else's.

We have to remember, Dad. You have to remember this, these times with Craig. Goddammit Dad, you can't forget him!

We walk outside to hear "Taps" played in Craig's honor, but the Bugle Corps doesn't show. No one knows what to say. Beau stands still, completely checked out of the proceedings. Ten years ago, he would have mitigated the situation. He would have driven to find the sheriff and wrung his neck.

Nora, in an act of great solitary courage, addresses the confused crowd.

"The service is over and we thank you all for coming. Your support means the world to me. Craig is with us."

She hangs her head and reaches for Beau's hand. It hadn't occurred to him to reach for hers. I want to kill him now. Trade him in for Craig. *The wrong person is dead,* keeps repeating in my head.

A handful of people join us back at Beau and Nora's condo. We nibble on carrots dipped in French dressing, courtesy of Trish's trip to Publix. At some point she had gone back and gotten a cake too.

Kathy bought some Bud Light, which was Craig's favorite beer.

A light bulb goes out over the kitchen sink. Beau finds a new one, and I get on the counter to replace the burned-out one. For some reason, I can't do it. My fingers are shaking. Lee hops up on the counter to help.

"It goes this way," I say.

"No, this way," he argues.

"You are still Dr. No after all these years!"

Kathy, in a moment of great comic relief, says, "How many Bercaws does it take to change a light bulb?"

Everyone howls with laughter.

"Three, apparently," I answer.

People go back to their beer and celery sticks. My father walks over to Kathy and puts his arm around her. His face is distorted, the way it always is when a pronouncement is forthcoming. The way he is hedging, grinning and blinking all at once, I can tell this will be a doozy.

"Well," he says, squeezing Kathy as tightly as a python, "how does it feel to be an only child?"

CHAPTER NINETEEN

THE BRAIN INSTITUTE
GAINESVILLE, FLORIDA

It is 2008 and forty-three-year-old me is worried about seventy-year-old Beau navigating my house in Vermont. I hear him at night trying to find the bathroom and peeing on the floor. He also seems to have lost interest in puzzles, and prefers to lie on the couch and watch television all day. I give him a job sorting Tinker Toys in David's room.

"Dad, put all the same colors together and wrap them with a rubber band."

He nods and begins to work. I leave him alone to finish.

An hour later, he hasn't come back downstairs. I take David up to check on Beau's progress. He is still sorting and rubber-banding.

David reaches into the Tinker Toy bin to retrieve a few stray pieces. Beau slaps his grandson's hand away.

"NO!" my father says harshly.

He has forgotten these are David's toys. Moreover, he's forgotten that he doesn't hit. After the physical abuse Beau suffered under Berc's hands, he swore to never strike his own children. He told me this when I accused him once of being a terrible father. "Not hitting you," Beau said, "was proof otherwise."

David goes from shocked to hysterical in two seconds. Beau goes back to sorting Tinker Toys. I retreat to find Nora.

"He's changing," I say, dancing around the subject as I was taught to do.

"Yes," she admits.

"It's here."

"I don't know, Nan. It may be depression."

My father may very well be depressed, but far more worrisome to me now is his declining cognitive skills. If anything, he is sad because he can't think well anymore—and he's aware of the slippage. He is worried, I can tell, which makes me worried.

Cousin Nancy had recently sent me a copy of letter that Berc had sent all his sons, back in 1960. She found it in her father Woodson's things after declining health—both mental and physical—sent him into a nursing home. The letter shed greater insight into our family history of obsession and depression.

> I don't like to write this, but I think you need it. And I have been putting off writing about our own family history, some of which is not good at all. As for my grandfather, George Washington Bercaw, he died in the Kentucky State Asylum. Of what I do not know as they did not keep records in those days like they do now. But I have heard my father say he never was much and he never had much to do with him. As for Grandmother Bercaw, she died insane in the same Asylum. First she was there about 5 years, then she recovered enough to get out, got pregnant, got child birth fever (they say), threw her baby down a well (I heard when about 4 or 5 years old), then back to the asylum for years until she died.
>
> As for my own father, he had digestive troubles, and was sensitive and nervous. He and my mother quarreled. In 1921, I was called home by my mother. There I found my father in bed with his throat and wrists slashed but not seriously. He was not normal, of course, and very depressed. After a few days I took him to a sanitarium in Atlanta which proved to be a sobering-up place for alcoholics. I stayed around a couple of days to see that my father got more used to the place. One day I took him for a walk in the sun, during which he asked me to kill him....

My grandmother made copies of every letter she and Berc ever wrote and received, and filed them in boxes by sender, date and year. The boxes were in the den at the farm, as accessible to readers as the books on the shelves. When she died, each son got everything he had ever sent to, and received from, Grandmother and Berc.

Nora told me that she had posed the "Alzheimer's vs. Depression" issue to Dr. Kenneth Heilman, professor and practicing neurologist at the University of Florida. Beau and Ken had been classmates in medical school at the University of Virginia. Then they met again in Gainesville, when Beau was a research fellow after we came back from the Philippines.

When Beau had started feeling "weird," as he described it to Nora, he requested that they visit Ken. Besides, it was best not to let anyone in Naples hear about Beau's issues. I imagined my father thinking "malpractice lawyers would have a field day" with a neurologist who might have had Alzheimer's disease while treating patients with the same.

Dr. Heilman was unable to confirm—or deny—any diagnosis, even after an MRI and the longest neurology exam on record. Not surprisingly, Beau had aced the mechanics of the test. He'd given the same physical exam upwards of eight times a day for forty years. He could count backward by seven even if he were in a coma. Whether Beau was in the initial stages of Alzheimer's disease was impossible to decipher. If the disease was there, he was outsmarting it.

We don't know what is wrong with Beau, other than being a Bercaw.

A year after their visit to Vermont, I go to Naples to take care of Beau while Nora has minor surgery and has to stay in the hospital. Beau needs a companion while she is away.

For the entire first day after my arrival my father hugs me every time he sees me come around a corner.

"Gal, it's so good to see you!"

These hugs are long, drawn-out, two-handed embraces—quite unlike the sideways, one-armed versions he used to give.

I feed him. I clean up his accidents. I let him eat Skinny Cow Ice Cream Sandwiches. I temporarily lose him in the grocery store when he strikes out on his own to find them. I nap when he naps.

I take him on daily visits to see his wife at the hospital, and stop him from calling her every five minutes when he's not there. I get the newspapers before he wakes up so he won't wander outside alone.

I hear him on the phone with a gold coin dealer one morning.

"I don't have any money anymore," Beau dejectedly tells the salesman. Then he hangs up. It's not his money that has dwindled, it's his mind.

While Beau watches a baseball game that afternoon, I walk into his den and eye the wall of supplements he used to take—bookcase after bookcase of pills with names like "Memoral" and "Sharp Mind," along with the standard vitamins and minerals. All brutal reminders of how valiantly he had fought to stave off this disease that none of us is naming. It seems symbolic that they are all past their expiration dates.

I rest my hand on the gun cabinet on my way out. *Not gonna need any of you, either.*

Every morning, I enlist Beau to walk to the local coffee shop with me. The only thing he says on these walks is "The hibisci are in full bloom."

Every time he says it, I ruminate on whether the plural of hibiscus is, in fact, hibisci. I feel better thinking about innocuous things than the gravity of the situation.

On my final day in Naples, we take one last walk together. As we start out, Beau is on the inside, closer to the curb. But a moment later, he takes my arm and leads me to the inside, like the gentleman he is—putting himself in the position closer to passing cars. He still knows how to protect me. Instinct trumping reason.

Beau doesn't mention the hibisci on this walk, though they are still blooming. I notice his gait is off, and for a second I think he might be having a stroke.

"Are you OK, Dad? You're walking funny."

"I'm just trying not to step on the cracks," he says, perfectly seriously.

I giggle. *He thinks he's a boy again! Maybe he's back on the farm, or walking the halls of the University of Virginia. Or maybe he's testing his own gait's agility.*

As we pass a particularly flourishing hibiscus tree, my father turns to look at me. *That look.* The one that means something big is coming.

"Gal," he says. "I sure appreciate you coming down to take care of me." His voice quivers at the end.

I compose myself long enough to say, "It was a pleasure, especially after all you have done for me. Besides, you don't need so much taking care of."

As we walk on, my father repeats this fixation every few minutes —with the same quiver in his voice in the exact same place. But each time, my emotions get bigger and my response gets shorter, until I am the one Alzheimer's disease has rendered speechless.

CHAPTER TWENTY

PULAI SPRINGS RESORT
JOHOR BAHRU, MALAYSIA

My whiter-than-white, five-year-old son, David Beauregard, is swimming in a blue resort pool in southern Malaysia with a beautiful brown Muslim boy named Ahmed. Holding hands is the only way they communicate their affection for each other. They zoom down the waterslide together with great velocity. They laugh and run back to the top to do it over and over again. It is 2010. I am forty-four.

I imagine my seventy-two-year-old father back in Florida commenting on the scene.

"He's just like you, Gal."

In reality, Beau's brain is drifting out to sea. I have run away to Asia, yet again, to be near what he is forgetting.

"Then he's just like you too, Dad," I say to the same South Seas breeze that once drifted through my nursery window in Angeles City, and Beau's in Manila.

David isn't a Filipino, like my father and I pretend to be by birthright. But he is a Virginian by legacy and birth. His skin is so translucent that his blue blood shines right through it. He bruises so easily that I have to stop myself from thinking he has leukemia.

I look over at Ahmed's mother. She is in the shade, covered from head to toe in a burqa. She doesn't feel me looking at her and doesn't return the gaze. I glance down at my uncovered legs getting pinker and more freckled by the minute even though I have 50 SPF sunscreen lathered on every inch of my body. I should cover myself in the interest of health and modesty.

Allan is sitting next to me, reading a book and napping at the same time. David's arrival surprised Allan enough for him to question my faithfulness. Before my Grandmother died and we moved to Virginia, I hadn't wanted children. I was afraid more than anything. One night, I changed my mind and I got pregnant then and there.

After we had the very first ultrasound, I sent the image to my father with a note that said, "It's a Bercaw." You could see my baby's big lips already.

I am more like my father now than ever. He took pictures of every place he traveled and showed them off in slideshow parties for his doctor friends. I would sneak out of my bedroom for a glimpse of what he had seen while he and my mother were away.

There was one picture of him that I can never get out of my head. My mother must have taken it from the window of the back seat of an Indian cab: Beau standing on the hood of a taxi in New Delhi and holding a big brass tray over his head. Thousands of Indians, and cattle, are looking up at him. Beau is pretending to be Moses; the tray is the Ten Commandments; the Indians are the Red Sea. Beau was trying to get to the Holy Land of the Taj Mahal Hotel, but half of Delhi was blocking the route.

"Did it work, Beau?" someone called out.

"Like a charm," my father said. He loved an admiring audience of oddballs—whether it was Indian pedestrians, Filipino pythons or his fellow Floridian physicians. But what he loved more than anything was making life better for his neurology patients.

Beauregard did not suffer fools gladly—especially when other people were in pain. He joined the Republican Party immediately after he witnessed Robert Kennedy strutting around Clark Hospital as if it were a cocktail party for him, ignoring the wounded and smiling for television cameras.

For thirty years I tried to understand my father, but I caught a rare glimpse into the inner workings of his mind one afternoon.

We were in Virginia visiting my grandmother in her nursing home, a few years before she died. After saying goodbye to her, we passed the open door of another resident. My father looked in, on physician's instinct, and I followed his lead.

A spastic middle-aged man was toppled over in his wheelchair. Beau calmly picked him up and put him back in the chair. They started conversing. I couldn't understand a single word the other man was saying.

Brtltm, spushc, huggle, muck....

My father introduced himself, and asked what the man's name was. I couldn't decipher it. But my father listened intently and laughed frequently as the man spoke.

"Did you hear that?" my father said. "Bruce spent his younger days working in his family's grocery store in rural Virginia. They're all gone now, so he's here."

I nodded to Bruce, and he said something back and then launched into a story about the old days, or at least I think he did. I had no idea what he was saying. I couldn't make out one word. Drool was pouring out the corner of Bruce's mouth as he spoke.

Brtltm, spushc, huggle, muck....

"Isn't he funny?" My father said, patting Bruce on the back. "You are a good ol' boy, working hard at your family store. Making everyone laugh in the aisles, I bet."

Bruce beamed up at my dad from his wheelchair for a long while before using his hand, curled up from cerebral palsy, to push the button to make his chair move forward into the hall.

"Bruce, wait," my father called after him. "Let me take a picture of you with Gal."

What I had learned in those few minutes is that my father had no interest in speaking with those for whom communication was easy. Those kinds of people use words frivolously. Bruce earned every word he spoke. He deserved to be heard and understood.

The older my father got, the more he used his camera to express emotion—taking your picture meant that he cared about you. The more he took, the deeper the affection. If he uttered the words, "that's a great one," it meant he was very pleased with his subject indeed.

One day Beau just stopped using his camera. He forgot that it mattered to him. From then on, I started taking pictures of everyone and everything. I was picking up where he left off—keeping him alive by taking on more of his traits.

I wished Beauregard could see me now—trying to get a slideshow-worthy picture of David and Ahmed, the two of them having the time of their lives without the burden of words. Water their common language.

I try to get closer to the boys, who are running here and there. Ahmed's mother looks at me as I pass. I notice that her mouth is significantly deformed, much more dramatically than a cleft palate. The right side of her lips are twisted up, down and all around. A few teeth are permanently exposed. She takes good care of them. They are white and shiny even though they are pointing in various directions. The left side of her mouth seems normal. It is like she had a stroke on top of a birth defect.

I wonder if she can speak at all, let alone in English. She points to her son hugging mine, and nods.

I know exactly what she means.

CHAPTER TWENTY-ONE

NIRWANA RESORT
BINTAN, INDONESIA

I wake up early to finish reading *The Dead Hand*, a novel by Paul Theroux, about the mysterious death of a ten-year-old Indian boy in Calcutta. Why am I reading this? I hate books in which children die. I am forty-four and my father has a death sentence. I guess I have to prepare myself, as his child.

Beau is in the mid-stages of Alzheimer's. The transformation is underway, although Nora has kept the details to a minimum. His dignity and privacy are more important than his incontinence and confusion. She does tell me that he has been fainting and falling down a lot—scary considering his size. He naps off and on, but still gets excited about Virginia football games.

To shake off thoughts of Theroux's book and my father's decline, I walk around the grounds of the Nirwana Resort, which is billed as "the Cheery Family Hotel."

We had come to Bintan, Indonesia because it was a one-hour ferry ride from Singapore where Allan has taken a teaching position for the year. Besides, this Cheery Family Hotel boasted an impressive swimming pool—actually, a series of four interconnected pools— with bubbles and rocks and plants. But most impressively, when you were in it, the pool seemed to stretch into the South China Sea.

We had been in Malaysia the month before. I wanted to see all the countries near Singapore, especially the ones with the best views of the ocean. We could have traveled here by Air Garuda Indonesia, Beau's favorite airline, but I wanted to be in the water, not the sky.

Back from the walk, I take David to the pool. Allan stays behind to find out about our ferry ride home that afternoon. He will pack up the room and leave our bags with the bellman. Is that what they call him? No, it's something different. Porter, maybe. It could even be "boy."

David and I sit down on the lounge chairs near the center of the pool, and his nose starts to bleed. I retrieve a napkin from the pool restaurant and give it to him to hold in place. Do you hold the bridge of the nose or the nostril area? Such a simple thing, yet no consensus amongst the medical community.

My back is to the pool. A sound, a movement, something, makes me turn around. I think it is someone running past me. Why running? I stand up and look.

I see a boy of Asian origin, approximately six or seven years old, lying on the deck in his blue swimsuit. The suit goes from his neck to his knees and is zipped in the front. Goggles are around his neck.

He is unconscious. A handful of people are around him. One of them is his mother with another very young child in her arms. I walk the short distance from the chair (leaving David behind to hold his nose) to do something. What will I do? Other people are moving quickly. I freeze.

A pool attendant—there are no lifeguards—begins CPR with short, slight chest compressions appropriate for a child. The mother drops to her knees beside her son and begins praying. I look around for her baby. Who took it? Is the father here too? Then I look back at the attendant working on the boy.

I point to my mouth—thinking the attendant needs to add mouth-to-mouth resuscitation to his chest compressions. But he is not looking at me. Should I drop down and push him out of the way? Should I give the boy a tracheotomy, like Beau taught me in the Puerto Rican rain forest? But the boy is not choking, he's drowning—or has he drowned? What is the process of dying by water once you are out of the water? Why is it only drowning and drowned? What is the time in between?

We are in that time.

The pool attendant begins mouth-to-mouth. Within two or three breaths, the boy vomits. *Clear the airway now*, I try to will into the attendant's head. But he knows what he is doing. Besides, I can't recall the procedure. Three compressions followed by two breaths?

A German woman in the pool starts screaming "turn him on his side" as she makes her way to the scene. She is correct. The vomit needs to be cleared from the boy's mouth. The attendant does that, and then resumes his CPR efforts.

"Keep him on his side!" the woman shouts.

No! I think. The boy needs continued resuscitation, which can't be performed on his side. But I say nothing. The attendant continues his work.

The mother screams for an ambulance in very good English, and pauses to say, "Be strong, be strong," to her son. She says his name over and over again. I can't make it out. Is it Justin? They are native English speakers of Asian origin.

Filipinos?

The boy's eyes open, but don't blink. They are glazed over. Where is he? Here or gone? He vomits again. The attendant puts his finger in the boy's mouth and clears it. I can't remember if vomit is a good sign — or just a reflex.

The German woman is still repeating, "Put the boy on his side," and she gestures for one of those devices that pump air into the mouth for you. This woman is annoying. She's distracting. I want to call her a dumb-dumb and tell her that old-fashioned mouth-to-mouth works. But I am reticent because that is how Beau raised me. Now, in a moment of crisis, I can't function.

I know about lambs' brains, the Heimlich maneuver, Alzheimer's, Parkinson's, the Taj Mahal and the Great Pyramid of Giza. I can speak Spanish, Swahili and Korean. But right now I can't recall how to do CPR, even though I have taken lessons in my adult years—

of my own volition. Why couldn't my father have made CPR a priority over sleep apnea and snakebites?

Beau was the author of an article in the journal *Geriatrics* titled "When Loss of Consciousness Is Not Caused by Epilepsy." I remembered reading it when I was eleven.

> The ordinary faint is perhaps the most frequent cause of a transient loss of consciousness. It occurs in response to an emotional or a physical stimulus that results in vasodilation, which theoretically is to prepare the individual for flight or fight. The blood pools in the extremities and venous return to the heart is inadequate, with secondary decline of cardiac output and cerebral blood flow.

Four hotel employees arrive with a backboard and quickly put the boy (on his side) on the board. The mother's younger child mysteriously is back in her arms again. Had the baby been there the whole time? Should I offer to take the child? Before I can say anything, the attendants are running with the boy toward the hotel. Why had they stopped CPR to transport him? You stop for two reasons: he is breathing fine, or he's never going to breathe again.

How did my father endure a lifetime of medical emergencies? Death showing up every single day for decades? One flash encounter with the Grim Reaper and I will never be the same again.

I turn toward David, who is still sitting on the lounge chair holding the tissue to his nose. Has he seen everything? He is very quiet. How long has it been? Thirty seconds or five minutes?

I hold David tightly. The German woman and her husband walk past.

I ask, "Is the boy going to be all right?"

She answers, "No, didn't you see his eyes?"

Her husband says, "My wife is a midwife. They should have been listening to her."

A midwife? Surely she knows about life and death. I squeeze David tighter and say, "Pray, pray, pray."

Allan arrives at the pool. The attendants carrying the boy had whizzed passed him. He saw the mother running behind.

I try to explain what I had witnessed, but I can only cry. I see one of the attendants return to the pool area with the backboard and point. Allan goes to speak with him. I watch them from a short distance while I hold David, who says, "I'm glad I know how to swim."

Allan gives me the thumbs up while he speaks with the man. I burst into sobs and cling to David.

"He's OK, David. He's OK."

I notice that most of the other vacationers are already back into their books and tanning. How can anyone return to normal? My sobbing reaches epic proportions.

David clings to me tightly, "Don't worry, Mommy, don't cry."

All I can think is that I want my daddy here—to fix the little boy and me. The drowning makes me miss Beau in ways I never expected.

Allan rejoins us. The man said that the boy was fine. But Allan thinks the way in which he said it was strange. Was it just a cultural difference? Or was the man told to tell everyone that the boy would be fine? Allan is unsure, but we want to believe the boy is OK—that CPR worked, which is why they stopped administering it.

All I know for sure is that I want to get as far away from this pool and Bintan, Indonesia as quickly as possible. We take David back up the stairs to the Cheery Family Hotel, where there is no trace of the emergency that flashed through minutes ago. Our ferry back to Singapore is scheduled for 2 p.m., but it's only 10 a.m. Allan tries to get us on an earlier ferry, to no avail. He says he is going to shop for presents for David and me, but I tell him that I have all the memories of this place I can handle.

The Indonesian dancers and the complimentary juice drinks are lined up to greet the next busload of guests. David helps himself to one of the juice drinks. They all feature plastic mermaids and mini-parasols. David picks out his tiny umbrella and prances around the lobby singing, "It's raining, it's pouring, the ol' man is snoring."

I sit down and watch the koi swim in the lobby pond. I try to stop the tears from falling out of my eyes, but water does as it pleases on this and every day. The koi seem to think that my tears are food and congregate near me. Once they realize that what is dropping into their pond is more of the same, they scatter. I have let them down, as well as that boy.

I should be in Florida helping my dad and Nora.

The water around Bintan, as we pull away on the ferry, is violent even though there is no storm. The captain advises us to stay seated and to use the bags if we experience "discomfort." Several people do.

Just as we reach the midpoint between Indonesia and Singapore, the ocean settles down. But my tears are like tsunamis. I replay the scene over and over again in my head.

Had the boy drowned or not? Beau would know. He would tell me.

Perhaps this is why my father was obsessed with Asia and the mind: you never really understand what is happening in either. The only sure things in either hemisphere of the world—or the brain—are fluid and death.

CHAPTER TWENTY-TWO

ANGKOR WAT

SIEM REAP, CAMBODIA

Our plane lands in Siem Reap and I feel opposite things at once. The same effect my father always has on me. This is a place of great joy and great suffering. It is 2010 and the country is struggling to recover from the genocide that took place here in the late '70s.

We have come to make a video for a nonprofit non-governmental organization based in Singapore that is building schools for Cambodian kids. Actually, Allan is making the video. David will play with the children.

I am here to remember what my father has forgotten.

Beau used to tell me, obsessively, about Pol Pot and the Khmer Rouge when they came to power in 1975. In addition to killing his countrymen, Pot was systematically destroying Angkor Wat. Built on the orders of King Suryavarman II in the early 12th century, Angkor Wat was made to honor Vishnu—Beau's favorite Hindu god—as well as the Khmer civilization. Centuries later, as the Khmer people converted to Buddhism, so too did portions of Angkor.

Beau explained to me how the expansive, finely detailed temples and bas-reliefs were made largely of sandstone and took thirty years to finish. Angkor is shrouded in mystery, he said, and overgrown vegetation. Experts believe it was made in the shape of the mythical Mount Meru—the home of the great Hindu god Brahma—with the central quincunx symbolizing the five peaks of the mountain.

The walls and moat are meant to represent the surrounding mountain ranges and ocean.

"Angkor faces west," Beau said passionately, pointing at the temple in a coffee table book he bought to further my studies. "Hindus believe this is the direction toward the afterlife."

"If the Americans hadn't bailed on the Vietnam War, Cambodia wouldn't have had Pol Pot," Beau had informed me.

I had no idea what he was talking about. I was just a kid who had learned, at school, about Hitler and the Holocaust—details of which caught me off guard and overwhelmed me. Beau told me plenty about the Japanese atrocities during World War II. I figured it was my duty to share my findings with him about the Germans.

"Dad," I said, right when he walked in the door one evening. "You are not going to believe this. You'd better sit down."

"What is it?"

"Well, there was another really bad guy. Worse than Pol Pot, I think. His name was Hitler and he tried to kill all the Jewish people in the world. He put them in gas chambers. Dad, can you believe how horrible that is?"

He put his arm around me. "I did know about that, Gal."

"What?" I said, shocked. "And you didn't tell me?"

I ran into my room. How could Beau have gone on and on about Chairman Mao and Pol Pot, and Castro too, but leave out Hitler? It didn't make sense.

Lying in my bed, I tried to think if we had any Jewish friends. Why weren't we inviting people with numbers on their wrists over to dinner? Were there none left? There weren't any Jewish students where I went to school. I remembered, though, that Beau's good friend Mike Dalton was Jewish. My dad adored Mike. Did they talk about Hitler?

I was certain that my father would be horrified to hear about the amount of suffering that took place in Auschwitz and other camps like it. But he hadn't even flinched. If he had known, why hadn't he been the one to tell me?

Beau had shown me pictures of children with horrendous neuro-logical deformities: myelomeningocele, also known as spina bifida; hydrocephalus, or water on the brain; and elephantiasis.

Beau had taken me to see an old-fashioned medical museum where deformed fetuses floated in jars. He had shown me pictures of the stacks of skulls that Pol Pot left in his wake. Why had he chosen to leave out the gas chambers?

I heard my father coming down the hall. His footsteps stopped at my door. He didn't come in. He talked to me with the door closed. He often did this, and I have no idea why except that he was a stickler for personal privacy.

"Gal, what I worry about is all the suffering that doesn't get as much publicity. The parts of wars people don't talk about, or don't agree with because they're socialists or part of the liberal media."

He paused. I stayed silent.

"Gal, you have no idea how terrifying the world is. The Holocaust is well known. One day I'll tell you about the North Vietnamese and what they did to people. I saw it on my operating table in the Philippines."

He walked away. *Dear God,* I prayed, *help me understand my dad and war. I'm not sure whose side I am supposed to be on anymore. I'm really scared. I think my father might be insane. Or else I am. Give me a sign.*

The next day, Beau left a book next to my bed, *When Hell Was in Session* by Jeremiah Denton. It is the true story of the torture Denton endured as a POW for seven years in Hanoi—four of those years in solitary. I race through the book from start to finish without stopping or eating.

One scene riveted me more than any other: Denton has been asked to speak at a press conference full of North Vietnamese officers and civilians. If he makes any attempt to communicate the hellish conditions of the camp, the punishment afterward would be un-bearable. On the spot, he comes up with a brilliant plan:

I gazed dully around the room, as though in a daze. The blinding floodlights made me blink, and I suddenly realized that they were playing right into my hands.

I felt my heart pounding; sweat popped out on my forehead; the palms of my hands became slippery. I looked directly into the camera and blinked my eyes once, slowly, then three more times, slowly. A dash, and three more dashes. A quick blink, slow blink, quick blink.

T...O...R....

A slow blink...pause; two quick ones and a slow one; quick, slow, quick; quick.

T...O...R...T...U...R...E....

I had recently found a postcard my father had written to his mother from Hong Kong in 1993, in which he commented exclusively on the status of free enterprise there.

Leave Hong Kong for Singapore tonight. HK has changed from 1966. Almost no junks or rickshaws. The people thriving and prosperous—too busy to worry much about the change in government from England to Red China in 1997. This city a great example of unfettered free enterprise—lowest prices in Asia with a thriving economy as opposed to ours. The dollar worth little here now.

I was pretty sure that I was the only kid receiving and reading *National Review* and Milton Friedman. I certainly didn't tell my friends, who were tuned into *Happy Days,* nor did I tell them that my father was hoarding huge tins of food and gold coins under the king-sized bed he shared with my mother. He also had shotguns and handguns of all sizes in his closet. When I was rummaging around in there once, looking for a rogue Snickers bar, I found a book called *The Kama Sutra*. I was beyond certain that my parents did not do what the pictures suggested. I dismissed it as research from a more primitive time before brains, as well as the free market, ruled.

"What kind of food is in those tins, Dad?" I asked.

"Basic provisions. Gal, if this country gets into a Bay of Pigs situation again, we'll have food when others may not."

My mother seemed unruffled by these realities. She came from a highly decorated military family too. My great-great-great uncle, Admiral Presley Marion Rixey, M.D., also a graduate of UVA's Medical School, was the personal physician to Presidents McKinley and Roosevelt, and the Surgeon General of the United States Navy. Admiral Rixey attended to McKinley after he was shot, and was the one to declare the president dead. Later he had traveled to review the creation of the Panama Canal with Roosevelt, and was mentioned frequently in the president's letters.

> U.S.S. *Louisiana*
> At Sea, November 20, 1906
>
> This is the third day out from Panama. We have been steaming steadily in the teeth of the trade wind…a tremendous sight to see the work on the canal going on…. We spent the three days in working from dawn until long after darkness—dear Dr. Rixey being, of course, my faithful companion….

Gentility was passed down through Rixey lineage they way depression was passed down to Bercaws.

Now I am in Siem Reap, and Cambodia's ancient splendor and tragic history are reminiscent of Beau's brain: two noble places eroded by a merciless, homegrown enemy.

Beau had visited Angkor Wat in 2001, at age sixty-four—the realization of a lifelong dream to see the majestic site. While here, Beau purchased a huge temple rubbing for me: an image of Shiva riding Garuda in some kind of victory parade.

Allan, David and I get picked up at the tiny rural airport in a minivan. We bump up and down on dirt roads, the way Beau and I had done in Kenya more than two decades earlier. Monkeys occasionally run out in front of the van. The driver doesn't slow down for them. Although we have our seatbelts on, I put my arms around David.

"This is the home of an ancient and great civilization," I tell David, holding back my tears. I am in some sort of incredible time machine looking at Beau's memories through my own eyes—speaking his words to my son.

We pass motorcycles piled high with chicken coops, lumber and families. We pull into the Tara Angkor Hotel, where the staff greets us by putting their hands together and bowing. We return the gesture. A porter takes our luggage because our ride to dinner is waiting out front. Tara, I recall, is the Hindu goddess for courage and compassion. She hears the cries of beings in misery.

"Mr. Million, The Flying Tuk-Tuk Driver," as he calls himself and as it reads on his crazy machine, welcomes us into the rickshaw that he drives with his motorcycle. He moves in and out of traffic and delivers us to an upscale restaurant that specializes in Cambodian food. The rest of the video crew meets us there, as does the school's Cambodian superintendent, Ung Savy.

We dine on Amok curry, lemon fish soup and lots of rice. I ask Savy if he would be willing to tell us what it was like when the Khmer Rouge ran his country. It will help us understand the state of education in Cambodia, I say, and what the schools are up against.

"But first," I say, channeling my father back at Mr. Tan's restaurant more than three decades ago, "let us tell you how honored we are to be here."

We toast to Savy, who begins to tell us how many in his family were killed—some of whom starved to death—during the period when Pol Pot tried to create an agrarian society. The educated were the first to die—frequently tortured to death. That is why there are no teachers or doctors in Cambodia, Savy says. A generation of enlightenment was eradicated.

I look over at David, worried that this discussion will frighten him. His head is on the table and he is asleep. I remember my brother at Mr. Tan's restaurant many years ago and put the napkins on David's shoulders to keep him safe from the mosquitoes that are coming through the open windows.

I gaze at Savy with tears in my eyes, as he continues to tell us the story of his country and his own family. I think of Beau and all the horrors of the world that he tried to warn me about. I can't believe I am in Cambodia now hearing the stories firsthand.

I watch Savy, the way Beau once fixated on Mr. Tan.

"The man who killed my family is my neighbor now."

No one knows what to say. I think to myself, *Why don't you kill him?* I suppose everyone at the table is thinking it—except Savy. He wants no more killing in Cambodia.

Surely Beau would understand that sentiment. So why was he in favor of death over Alzheimer's? All Beau ever did was fight for life. Why give in to a predator of any kind, be it Pol Pot or dementia?

I will not kill my own father for acquiring Alzheimer's.

Allan spends the next two days filming the students at the schools that an American woman, Jamie Amelio, started after meeting a little girl at Angkor Wat. When the girl asked for a dollar, Jamie asked what she needed it for and the girl replied that she needed it to go to school. Jamie visited the dirty, dilapidated, teacher-free school and decided to make a difference in the educational lives of Cambodian children. In the ten years since, with the help of friends in Singapore and Texas, she has built five schools and trained dozens of teachers. She also started the Food for Thought Program to feed the students when they arrive in the morning. I imagine that Beau would have had a huge crush on her.

While Allan works, David and I explore Siem Reap. Mr. Million takes us anywhere we want to go. We visit the Angkor National Museum and shop at the outdoor market. I give David two dollars to pick a souvenir. He chooses a stuffed salamander. I select a purse made out of a rice bag with, inexplicably, a blonde mermaid on it. I buy a statue of Garuda for my father.

We visit the Amelio School at the end of the second day and arrive just in time to hear Allan teaching the students to sing, "All You Need Is Love."

I look down at the T-shirt I'm wearing, which I bought in Singapore. It says "Love."

I sit on a tire swing to watch the filming. David sits on the bottom of the slide and sings along. It is so hot we can barely move. David's face is beet red. Mr. Million takes us back to the hotel so we can swim in the pool. We pass lots of Cambodians bathing in the river that runs through Siem Reap. It is muddy and motionless, a very unhealthy mix, my father would say if he were here.

But where he is, in Florida, Beau hardly says a word anymore. I am not entirely sure he would remember what cholera, dysentery and malaria are. His illness has erased his profession—and is beginning to wipe out the rest of him too. The build up of beta amyloid plaque in his brain is like a black plague. First one cell is affected and then another until the whole place is destroyed.

The next day, Mr. Million picks us up at 7 a.m. to drive us to Angkor Wat. He darts between dozens of buses filled with Japanese tourists to get us to the front of the entry gates.

"I didn't expect this," I tell Allan at the ticket window, where we pay $20 each in U.S. cash to visit the temples. "I guess the whole world knows about Angkor now. I thought it was just me and my dad."

The world knows about Alzheimer's too. Beau's pioneering interests are household words now. There is a whole association devoted to the cause.

Mr. Million speeds ahead of the other tuk-tuks. He is very devoted to us, as we are to him. Allan is going to give him film credit, as well as the brand-new sneakers he got in Singapore. Mr. Million's rate for unlimited travel is $10 per day. We double that fee.

As we round a corner for our first glimpse of Angkor, I hold my breath. My father prepared me for this all my life, just as he did Alzheimer's, and both have finally arrived. Angkor, like Beau's brain, is under a thick veil of haze.

Mr. Million lets us out at the main entrance and we cross a long bridge over the moat toward a structure that is a symbol of my life, as well as that of the Cambodians.

I grab David's hand. If he got lost here, I'm not sure we would ever find him. Angkor expands exponentially. It makes the Taj Mahal appear minuscule, and the Great Pyramid of Giza seem like basic architecture.

The swirls in Angkor's five spires are marked like a cerebrum. I feel like I am walking right into my father's head.

I find the place where the rubbing Beau gave me may have originated. Scenes of Vishnu riding Garuda are part of the outer gallery of "Vishnu conquering the Asuras." Asuras are demons, also known as the enemies of God. There are eight galleries in total, which form the rectangular gate around Angkor.

I wonder why this scene had captivated Beau before realizing the answer is obvious: Vishnu, with the help of Garuda, is *conquering* demons.

My father loved Asia, Hinduism and Buddhism for one reason: they provided something greater than Christian redemption.

They offered *reincarnation*.

In another lifetime, after lessons had been learned, Beau wouldn't turn into his father. His brain would be free to begin again and the cycle of dementia would end.

The morning before we are supposed to leave Cambodia for Singapore, we ask Mr. Million to take us to see the famed lake houses. After a short drive, we arrive in a vast open area where all the houses are on stilts but there is no water. These bamboo homes are tree houses without the trees, like the one I had as a kid. The Cambodians who live here climb down ladders to get to the ground.

"Where's the lake?" I ask.

"It hasn't come yet," Mr. Million says. He points at the dark clouds gathering. "Soon, it will be here again."

We are in Cambodia prior to the rainy season, which will soon turn this bone-dry land into an Asian Venice. For now, even the "floating kindergarten," which is written in English on a large houseboat, is grounded. Such a complicated country—there are two entirely different landscapes depending on the weather. And whichever one is present is the one in which Cambodians reside. They don't pray for rain when none is expected. They don't wish for sun when none is to come. They fish when water is present. They farm when land is at hand.

The wind picks up, and Mr. Million puts his Flying Tuk-Tuk in high gear to get us back to Siem Reap before the downpour. I watch the smiling survivors of the Khmer Rouge look up at the first drops of rain from their beached tree houses. One mother lifts her naked child from the bamboo deck and takes her inside.

I imagine myself blinking a message to Beau in Morse code.

A dash. A quick blink, slow blink, quick blink.

I...L...O...V...E...Y...O...U

CHAPTER TWENTY-THREE

JUNIPER VILLAGE MEMORY CARE
NAPLES, FLORIDA

Allan is offered a three-year contract to stay in Singapore. But Beau is getting worse in Florida. I can no longer pretend that I am nearer to my father by living in Asia. It is 2010—a year that is passing very slowly. I feel fifty but I am still forty-four. We decide to head home, refusing the offer of a lifetime. First stop is Naples.

Beau recognizes me after a few minutes. I suggest a round of Mad Libs after dinner.

"Dad, give me a plural noun. You know a person, place or thing with an 's' added at the end."

"Buzzards," he laughs. The word itself is so funny. Then, every time I ask for a noun, he says, "buzzard" or "buzzards," and laughs as if it were the first time. His reaction makes us laugh too.

Beau's harshness is greatly diminished, but so are his short-term memory and balance. He can still do long math in his head, but he can't remember who is the president of the United States—probably because Obama is a Democrat. A fact he doesn't want to remember.

A few months after Allan, David and I get settled back in Vermont, Nora needs me to return. Beau is in the hospital from falling and hitting his head. He is very confused.

"Nan, I think it's time we look for a safe place for him to live."

I can't breathe. But I know she is right. I book a flight to Florida. I call Kathy and she decides to come too. Nora has found a memory care facility near their home. She wants my approval. I don't tell her that I am supposed to kill Beau before this can happen.

Beau is home from the hospital when I arrive in Naples. It takes him a while longer to remember who I am. Finally, he says, "Hi, Gal." Then he asks me how many children I have.

Kathy and I play Mad Libs with Beau. I have to tell him what a noun or an adjective is over and over again. He can barely come up with a word, or any words, even after I explain what is needed.

I ask Kathy for a plural noun and she says "buzzards" to test him.

Beau looks up at her from his cereal bowl.

"Did you say 'buzzards'?" he asks very seriously.

"Yes."

Beau turns pale and stares back into his bowl. "Buzzards" seems to ring a faint bell, but he can't hear it. I ask him for a noun.

"Crow," he offers, sadly. He knows something is very wrong, too.

"Game over," I tell Kathy.

The next morning, on the way to tour Juniper Village, we stop at Barnes & Noble. Kathy and I want to postpone our arrival at the inevitable. We are not excited about touring the place where Beau will live out his days. While we are out, he is at home with an aide and has no idea where we're going. But I know Beau is ready for this step based on my rudimentary Mad Libs' neurological test—which he failed.

I ask Nora what happened to the brain in a jar that Beau used to have. She tells me she never saw it. She doesn't know what I am talking about. *What jar? Whose brain?*

"That must have been before my time," Nora surmises.

I briefly wonder if there ever had been a brain in a jar. Did I make it up to make sense of my father? No, my mother had seen it too. She was the one who told me that it was Berc's brain.

Once Beau met Nora, he no longer needed his father's brain in a jar. He had something and someone else to hold onto—for hope, instead of fear.

Nora, Kathy and I pull into Juniper's parking lot, and all I can see is a fence. My father will die if he has to live like a caged animal. He will become so depressed and lonely that he will curl up in his brand-new bed and pray for the end. Killing him might be the right thing to do.

Beau learned about mercy as a boy on the farm in Virginia. When unwanted kittens were born, his job was to put them in a burlap sack with a brick and throw them into the Rivanna River. It was kinder than letting them starve to death, he explained to me.

"But you love cats, Dad!" We always had one, or two, around our house.

"That why I had to kill those kittens, Gal. If you love something, you don't let it suffer. You put it out of its misery."

"Why couldn't you or Grandmother just buy them cat food?"

"It was war time, and we didn't have enough for ourselves and the farmhands."

"What about a few squirts of milk from the cows?"

"Gal, there was none to spare. There are things you don't understand about suffering. I have given you everything you've ever wanted. Spoiled you."

Sometime after our conversation about killing kittens, Beau took me to the Pinellas County Fair. I suppose I was seven or eight. My brother was too young to go with us. My father picked me up from school during lunch to take me. We walked right past the rides and cotton candy and midway games. I asked if I could try to win a goldfish, and Beau shook his head.

"Hurry, Gal, we only have an hour before I have to see patients again."

Beau bought two tickets for $1 each at a small booth.

"Go right in," the man said. "A few sights for sore eyes!"

I grabbed my father's hand as we went up a flight of stairs and into a dark room except for a light coming through two big glass windows. I stood up on the stool to peer inside.

The Fattest Man in the World was sprawled out across a huge round bed. He was watching TV in a huge diaper and not much else.

The edges of his gargantuan stomach seemed singed, as if they had been burned. I couldn't understand what I was seeing.

I looked at Beau, who just stared at the Fat Man for a long, long time. I couldn't figure out if he saw what I did. My father seemed to be far way, in a fairy tale, or a laboratory.

I studied the Fat Man too. He was watching a show that I had never seen. I wondered if Dad was considering taking the man home with us. I liked the idea if it meant I could watch more TV.

Or was my father plotting a way to drown the Fat Man and end his suffering? But the Fat Man wasn't starving to death. Maybe the opposite holds true. People eating themselves to death should mercifully be put out of their misery. It would take a lot of bricks and we would have to find a really deep part of the Rivanna.

Beau took my hand and led me to the next window. Inside, the Smallest Man in the World sat in a chair and stared back at us. This man's arms and legs seemed extra short, and his forehead was huge. Again, Beau was lost in the image. I thought I might throw up. I didn't understand what was happening on either side of the window. I figured there was something wrong with us too.

Maybe Beau had brought me there so the freaks could see the Filipino Bercaws.

"Gal, time to get you back to school and me back to the office."

"OK," I said, taking a big breath because I had to ask a question.

"Dad, do you think we should drown these people in the Rivanna River?"

"Quite the opposite," he said, smiling.

I shrugged, at home in his ambiguity. If the freak show was supposed to point out how spoiled I was in my own freaky life, then so be it.

I dare to ask another question.

"Dad, are you saying that I should be grateful that I'm not suffering like those two men?"

"No, Gal. I'm saying none of us can be happy when anyone is suffering."

Beau stopped at the fish ping-pong game and bought twenty balls. We tried to get them into one of the fifty or so bowls. I finally did and carried my goldfish back to the car like a trophy. The little creature swimming placidly in a plastic baggie offset the bewildering big man walking next me.

"What's her name?" Beau asked.

"Kitty."

Beau put his arm around me.

"Child of my heart," he said softly.

Sometimes Beau seemed sorry for his obscurity and complexity. Like he knew it was just too much for normal people. Yet, he didn't actually apologize. Because no matter how complicated his frame of mind, it had the side effect of improving yours too.

But now Beau's mind has turned on him.

Nora, Kathy and I walk into the administrative offices of Juniper Village. Gail meets us with a big smile on her face.

"Welcome," she says, escorting us to her office. She has two caged birds near her desk. The irony is a dagger in my heart.

Yes, I want to say, *welcome to this freak show, you caged animals, a place called Memory Care, which is code for You Actually Can't Remember Anything and We'll Make a Profit From It.*

My father wouldn't want me to think like this. Sarcasm is for lazy minds. Solutions are much harder to imagine. He would send me to my room. Instead, I will be relegating him to one here. While I am comforted by the fact that he had recommended this same route for his father four decades ago, I know Beau would rather be dead now than to die here later.

Gail brings us into her office and we sit around a table. I can't think of a question to ask her. I try to imagine Beau in this place, and I have to hold back my tears. *I will not cry*, I tell myself. *This is what's happening. Soldier on, the Death March is far from over.*

Gail starts telling us about what goes on at Juniper—which means "evergreen"—and how the residents enjoy themselves. Field trips to the zoo, clubs, holiday gatherings.

"The first week can be an adjustment, though," she says. "We recommend that Nora not visit him during that time."

My tears won't wait a moment longer. Nora is the reason Beau gets up in the morning. He is completely and utterly devoted to her. In his mind, he made a pact with the devil to love her.

That won't work, I want to say, but I can't articulate what I am thinking.

Gail could drown in the amount of water I am producing. If only I had a brick and a burlap bag. We could go down together.

Beau is the exception to every rule—except, of course, the rule of genetics. As a doctor, it didn't matter if his patients could pay him or not. He treated them no matter what, and consequently, they wanted to do things to repay him. In my youth, our house had been filled with carpenters, cleaners and mechanics working off their medical bills. Not because Beau asked them, but because they believed he was worth every penny.

We begin the tour of Juniper Village. Can any of these people outswim a gator with a boy on their chest? Did anyone here perform surgery on a lab rat they named Rodent E. Lee? Was this a place that could understand the nuances of a Hindu Christian who also became a Maragoli tribal chief? Did anyone here ever buy narcotics on the streets of Kathmandu to fight off a brutal sinus headache?

It doesn't matter anymore. It is time to stop fighting. I hang my head as we enter Cottage One. Gail shows us an empty room. Without décor or linens, it is so sterile. I think of Beau sitting in here alone wondering where his life and wife have gone. Because our DNA is so similar, I have come to believe that I can read his mind. He doesn't like it here. He would rather be dead. I laugh, remembering how he always said, "Better dead than red," as in Communist Red.

Gail introduces us to the social director, who is putting up the October calendar. She shows me how some of the residents have made turkeys by tracing their hands. I double over in laughter. She seems pleased. When my laughter turns into hysterical sobbing, Kathy escorts me back to the administrative offices.

"If she suggests that Beau should trace his hand to make a turkey, then God save her. Beau will give her the look, even in his diminished state."

I was referring to the look that has turned the fiercest ambulance-chasing lawyers into pillars of salt. Kathy nods. She knows.

Gail and Nora join Kathy and me in Juniper's administrative offices. Gail tells me that she knows it is not easy. She is the one I should shoot. But even if I did, Beau will still die in a place like this. Juniper is the River Styx. Gail is just the ferryman. We will pay her—or some other incarnation of Charon—a lot of money to escort Beau to the other side.

CHAPTER TWENTY-FOUR

FLETCHER ALLEN HOSPITAL
BURLINGTON, VERMONT

It is December 27, 2010, my birthday. I am finally forty-five. I call my father at Juniper because I know he won't remember to call me. My heart longs to hear him sing "Happy Birthday" and to say, "Your ol' dad sure loves you."

One of the Haitian aides in his cottage retrieves my father for me. I can hear him fumble with the phone—an apparatus he never much cared for in the first place.

"Hi, Dad, it's Gal."

"Hi, Gal."

"How are you doing?"

"I'm doing fine."

"Do you have a newspaper?"

"No."

"OK, I'll have one sent to you."

Silence.

"Dad, are you OK?"

"Yes."

"Are you sad?"

Silence.

"Dad, are you sad?"

"Am I sad?" He's puzzled by my question. "Well, I guess I'm sad I can't make love to Nora."

Final proof, as if needed, that Beau should be in Juniper. Never, ever, ever would he have said that to me if plaque weren't clogging up his brain.

"Can you watch the football games?"

"I guess so."

"Do you know what day it is?"

Silence.

"Is there anything you need?"

Silence.

What he needs is for me to kill him. To put him out of his misery. To drown him like an unwanted kitten on a farm. To put the dagger in his back, like the Little Mermaid should have done to the prince who forgot about her. I won't do it. I would rather kill myself.

"I love you, Dad."

"I love you, too."

He doesn't say it in the third person anymore. I would rather have his mind back than his first-person love. Now he says what he is feeling without a filter. I miss the uncertainty that defined my life.

I picture Beau lying in his bed at Juniper most of the day, staring at the ceiling fan. He gets up for meals, or if he is asked to go to the men's club meeting. He only does these things because he is a gentleman. He thinks meetings are stupid. Meals are worthy, though, especially if rice or fish are involved.

I ask Beau if they serve fish at Juniper.

"You are sending a fish?" he asks, confused.

"No, I am wondering if they feed you fish."

Silence.

I am talking to Beau as if he were an Orca "killer" whale at Sea-World and I was his trainer: Show me what you've learned, and I'll reward you! Meanwhile, you can swim in circles with your dorsal fin flopped over indicating your unhappiness, and your audience will pretend it means nothing. The flopped fin, your misery, is just the price of conserving the breed.

I am not sending Beau fish, but I will send him Butter Rum Life

Savers. Maybe the Life Savers will have the opposite effect. Perhaps he will choke on one and die. What we need now is Life Enders. I laugh at my absurd thought process, and then I start crying.

"Goodbye, Dad, I'll call you soon."

I hear him put the phone on the counter instead of on the hook. I hear one of the aides tell him that a football game is on TV before she hangs up the phone.

Two weeks before Beau moved into Juniper, his neurologist, Dr. Matthew Baker, brought up the subject of next steps. It was the first time Beau had actually been confronted, face-to-face, about his memory loss.

"Dr. Bercaw, what do you think is next for you?" Dr. Baker said.

Nora told me that Beau looked puzzled, as if he had been asked a riddle.

"Where do you think you should live?" Dr. Baker pushed.

"Home?" Beau might have been wondering if this was some sort new series of questions designed to assess a patient's neurological function.

"Dr. Bercaw, you have Alzheimer's and need special care now. I think you and Nora need to talk about this."

Beau went pale. He cried all the way home, asking Nora repeatedly, "Do you think I have Alzheimer's?"

Nora told him, "Oh, it's just a label. They need to explain your memory troubles to file the insurance."

By the late afternoon, thank God, he had forgotten what Dr. Baker had said.

I am secretly hoping Beau doesn't really have Alzheimer's disease. Maybe what he has is Bercaw's disease, in which eccentricity reaches such a degree that a Bercaw can no longer function in a non-Bercaw world. It might look like brain atrophy on an MRI, but it really means that the afflicted Bercaw is shrinking into himself.

It is happening to me, too. I can't remember a lot of stuff—and I don't know if it's because I am grieving over my father or if I'm in the early stages of Bercaw's disease. I am talking less. I'm sleeping more. These things are happening to me in the same way other people go bald.

I suggest my Bercaw theory via email to Dr. Baker. He says I might not be entirely off base.

> In certain neurological disorders, there seem to be pre-morbid personality traits, and I wonder if those genes are linked so closely that they cosegregate. There are several studies that show that certain neurotic traits are present in patients prior to developing AD. It makes sense that something so genetic has to begin years before the onset of the obvious symptoms.

I write to another one of my father's old colleagues, Dr. Michael Lusk, a neurosurgeon. Mike had arrived in Naples shortly after my father and Nora. Beau believed he was very talented, and was something of a mentor to his young friend. In gratitude, Dr. Lusk gave my father fantastic gifts, including an original Confederate shotgun from the Civil War. Beau had it framed and hung it over his desk. The same desk made in the Philippines that once was home to the contents of Berc's head.

A shotgun and a brain: the final prescription.

I ask Dr. Lusk, who had visited Beau in the hospital when he had a strange stroke-like spell a month or so before going into Juniper, if he would send me my father's last MRI results. I tell him that I don't want to bother Nora, but that the images might be helpful to me. I want to see inside Beau's head. I want to see the proof. And maybe peer into the future of my own brain.

Dr. Lusk writes back in the affirmative, and offers his condolences.

> I did go by to see Beau.... He did not seem to recognize me. It is quite sad. At least he seemed happy and not agitated. I agree with placement. Beau did not have any idea where or why he was in the hospital. I am so sorry that this has happened to your father. He was (is!) such a great man.

Beau's MRI results arrive a few days later. I can't look at them. I just fixate on this sentence in the accompanying results letter:

Moderate to severe atrophy and deep white matter chronic ischemic changes.

Since Beau's brain has diminished, my capacity for thought has too. The only thing tethering me to earth is my son. The child of my heart—who loves swimming and Asia—and seems to understand suffering the way my father did: *a thing to be respected.*

While I was pushing David in the stroller a few years back, a man who was missing a leg was walking in front of us. He must have been a new amputee, as he wore no prosthesis and used crutches. He was a young man. From David's point of view in the stroller, he had a good, close look at the stump. I wondered if it frightened or worried David, so we stopped and let the man get far ahead of us. I told David that sometimes people lose an arm or a leg but not to worry about it. They can do everything just fine and live great lives.

"Well," David said, "I hope it happens to me."

Then I had to explain to him why it might be best to keep our limbs if we can. He didn't seem convinced. *Oh, baby Beau, will you lose your mind like your grandfather?* The fear is growing in me that I will get Alzheimer's. I am Beau's clone.

Not only did my father and I have the same heads on our shoulders, but we had the same shoulders as well. We had witnessed each other's rotator cuff agony on many occasions. As a young swimmer, my shoulders were tested by the amount of time I spent pulling my body through the pool. When I hit my maximum pain capacity, my father took me for cortisone shots.

"Gal, you're like a racehorse," he said every time.

Sometime after that, we were skipping rocks from a train trestle on one of our camping trips. The action threw my father's right shoulder out of place. His pain was so great that he could barely utter instructions. Thirteen-year-old me was scared to death. All I could think was that a train would come before I could get him to the hillside.

"Gal, climb on my arm," he cried. "Pull on it with all your weight."

"Dad, can we get back to the side first?"

"No, do it now."

I grabbed onto his elbow and lifted my body weight onto his forearm. Both feet off the ground.

"Pull harder," screamed my father, blinded by pain.

I put my feet back and grabbed his upper arm and pulled down with all my might. Tears streaming down both our faces.

I heard a pop.

"Gal, you did it. You got my shoulder back in."

I think we celebrated with ice cream somewhere. Beau said he didn't need to go to a doctor, but I felt like I did.

After I graduated from college, an orthopedic doctor took one look at my shoulder and said that very little was holding it in place and that I needed rotator cuff surgery. My father told me not to worry, he would be there when I came out of the operating room.

My father stayed with me, demanding that the nurses bring me morphine whenever it wore off—not every four hours as prescribed. They did what he said, against the orders of the other doctor and the law. They knew Beau. He knew me.

Beau bought me a goldfish to look at so I could think about something else besides the pain. I stared at it day and night for two days, until I was well enough to go home. Nobody else remembers that goldfish, so I may have hallucinated it—remembering the goldfish "Kitty" from the freak show long ago.

Twenty-five years later and my left shoulder suddenly starts acting up again. I find an orthopedic doctor in Vermont and explain my swimming history. The long scar on my right shoulder surprises him.

"Before arthroscopic surgery, huh?" he comments.

He orders an MRI to get a better view of my tendons, and to make a decision about surgery.

I show up for the MRI in fine spirits, eager to get the results and know my fate. The techs help me lie down and slip my shoulder into the right spot.

"Have you been in an MRI before?" one of them asks.

"Yes," I say, jauntily. "I had one for some ear trouble a few years back. I was totally fine. I was raised around these machines. My father mortgaged our house to buy imaging equipment. An MRI is like home to me. Old hat, as it were."

They turn the machine on and slowly usher my head and body into the tight container. I am giddy to be in one of Beau's favorite devices.

Then suddenly I can't breathe. I push the emergency button. My flight-or-fight response is in full force.

"Are you OK?" one of the techs calls out.

"No, get me out of here now."

They pull me back out. I am in a full-blown panic attack and I don't know why. I feel rage and hatred toward this machine.

"What would you like to do, Nancy?" the tech asks me.

I want to tell her that I think my shoulder misses my father. But then they will send me right to the psych ward. I have to do this. I have to go back in and get this done. It may be tight inside but there are openings on either end. Jesus Christ, I used to be a great, fearless athlete. What the hell is the matter with me?

"Give me a moment to do some relaxation breathing," I say. After a few minutes have passed, I indicate that I am ready to go into the MRI again.

This time I push the panic button instantly and I know exactly why. This machine is a tragic reminder of what Dr. Beauregard Lee Bercaw has lost—his memory and his identity—and that I have lost him.

CHAPTER TWENTY-FIVE

JUNIPER VILLAGE MEMORY CARE
NAPLES, FLORIDA

When you see the Taj Mahal in person, you can't be certain that it is real. All you have ever known is a two-dimensional image. You cannot reconcile that picture with the real thing before your eyes. That is what it's like to be in my father's brain now.

I have pulled into Juniper on January 17, 2011, the same day an essay I wrote about Beau appears in the *New York Times'* Science section. Even though it is only 1 p.m., I have already received 200 emails about him and the article, titled "When All Isn't Enough to Foil Alzheimer's."

One of them is from a former employee of my father's back in the Largo days, thirty years ago.

> Your Dad pulled me out of the file room when I was 16 yrs. old and handed me a lab coat and whisked me away to make rounds with him. He said the most important lesson to learn was how to carry a hot coffee and walk at the same time. I am only 5'3" so keeping up with his strides wasn't so easy, but it was such a great experience. Your Dad to me is like one of the great old time movie actors who has such a persona, but is just a pussycat inside. If there is anything I can do to help you in any way or any questions let me know. I will be looking forward to your book about the famous Beauregard Lee Bercaw.

Another email is from Dr. Steven T. DeKosky, Vice President and Dean, and Professor of Neurology, at the University of Virginia.

> First, my condolences. I have been taking care of people with AD my entire career, and have no raft of survivors, as do my oncology colleagues. I knew your dad—I went to graduate school in neuroscience and psychology at UF and then to medical school there, and then moved back to do my residency in Gainesville after doing Medicine at Hopkins. Your dad was one of the senior neurologists in the state; I met him a few times at meetings, and he was a well-respected neuron (sic), with a mellifluous and wonderful voice, as I recall. When I read your piece in the Times, I wanted to send my sympathy and let you know that I remember him as I remember many of my own friends and patients—as remarkable people even during their illness.

I walk up to the chain-link fence that keeps Juniper's residents from walking away and getting lost. I put my hands on the wire, and look at the buildings inside. I close my eyes and go back to Huntsville, Alabama. Beau is standing next to me again. We are looking at the pool for a space to swim. I imagine his hand in mine, and inhale our shared courage from that day. We were outsiders then, wanting to get in. Now we are in and want back out.

I open my eyes and open the gate. I walk toward Beau's room. It has been two months since he became a permanent resident here.

My father is lying in his bed and looks up at me like I am the Taj. His eyes are as big as saucers. He says nothing. He knows who I am, I think, but the words seem dammed up. He grins and grimaces at the same time.

"Hi, Dad, it's me, Gal!"

He is still staring.

What does he see? Me as a kid, but with wrinkles? Maybe he thinks I am Grandmother.

Why does my little girl look like my mother? Where are we in space and time?

I don't have the best grasp on it, either. I am shutting down just as Beau is trying to reawaken. Where will we meet?

I hold up the Garuda statue I bought for him in Cambodia. It is so strange that a thing I got there is now here. We can't hold onto time, only evidence of times past.

"Garuda!" I say.

Beau nods awkwardly from his bed, still unsure of the situation.

"Yes, Garuda."

He doesn't care if we talk or not. He never did. I don't have to do some song and dance for him. I can use all my strength to hold back tears. He can devote himself to figuring out what the hell is going on.

Yet, somewhere in this mix of what each of us is trying to accomplish, I realize that I am the product of a life with him. He prepared me for this moment in time—for this eventuality—by filling my head with joy and tragedy in equal measure. Maybe Beau wasn't trying to stave off the disease. Maybe he was trying to get me ready for his certain demise.

Or maybe he was more worried about *me* getting the disease, and what he was fighting for all his life was *my* future—not his. Beau wanted to make me smarter, not to be a Bercaw, per se, but to stave off this Bercaw disease. He brought me up to be courageous and spiritual in the hopes that I could handle whatever came to pass. Whether purposely or not, he expanded my imagination, by reading books and seeing the world, so I could document the suffering of families like ours.

Beauregard Lee Bercaw raised me to believe in fairy tales and Hindu gods.

He raised me to see that a white American man born in the Philippines could become an African tribal chief.

He raised me to understand that kittens must drown sometimes, and that mermaids don't always have tail fins.

And now, everything that once occupied his head has been transferred to mine. There is nothing left to say.

I understand him.

One of the aides at Juniper decides she needs to communicate for us. She looks at me and then at my father, whose bed she has come to change. Two Bercaws connected by being lost in thought.

"You are twins," she says in a strong Haitian accent. "Come on, Dr. Beau, get up, your daughter is here. You should go on a walk."

I help Beau sit up, and put his sandals on. He uses the restroom, and then asks for his hat. He reaches out for my hand.

We take a walk around the courtyard, past the blooming hibisci that he loves. We find a row of chairs on a patio.

"I'll take the middle one," Beau says.

We look back from whence we had come. The sun is shining, but a slight cool breeze keeps the day from feeling India hot.

"It's a lovely day," Beau says.

"Especially when the breeze comes," I respond.

Beau turns to look at me again. He studies my face. He has not called me Gal, yet. He knows it's me, though. I think he is just trying to figure out what is going on with my face. The sun damage on my cheeks is very noticeable, as are the wrinkles near my ears and around my mouth. He used to buy me special creams in his natural-supplement phase.

I am looking back at him. His skin is very chapped. His face is blotchy. We both need to have a number of precancerous cells removed. We always do. We should not have been swimming all day in the summer sun in our youth. We are far too fair. He always tried to get me to put sunscreen on, but I refused. It made me look whiter than white.

Beau's sleeves are blood-stained. Nora has tried covering his arms in bandages, but it is no use. Beau wriggles his fingers below the bandages and scratches anyway. His doctor thinks the memory-preserving drug Beau is now taking is contributing to this obsessive-compulsive picking of his skin. The doctor may take him off of it, as it is probably no longer effectively curbing Beau's memory loss.

Thank God no one ever medicated Beau for showing signs of

OCD while he was a neurologist! Obsession made him very good at his job.

My father's teeth are pretty yellow. I don't think he is brushing them. He smells a bit yeasty, like he has been taking antibiotics and has acquired thrush. I smell like white wine. I am drinking too much wine these days, on top of two different kinds of antidepressants. Beau would chastise me if he knew.

We look back at the courtyard, away from each other. There is a nice wind chime hanging off the gutter at the edge of the patio. The breeze isn't strong enough to make it move. One of the other residents, a gentleman with a cane, is coming toward us.

"I'm confused," the man says upon arrival.

I look at my father, trying to read his face and mind. Beau puts his left hand up to his mouth, the way he always did when he was studying a situation. Gators, snakes, patients. For the first time ever, I can't tell what he is thinking—even by observing him closely. Thanks to Alzheimer's, what's in his head and what's on his face no longer match.

"I used to have a garage. Do you know where my garage is?" the man says.

Beau says nothing. He seems faintly annoyed. Not at the man's condition, of course. My father tried to help men like this guy all his life. But Beau is now part of the group of people formerly known as his patients—and it troubles him in a way he doesn't understand and can't express.

"No garages around here, I'm sorry," I say.

The man goes inside.

Beau and I go back to looking at the courtyard.

"Sure is a nice day," he says.

"Especially when that breeze comes," I add.

Beau turns to look at my face. I know he doesn't like what he sees. He is studying me very intently, like I am a Petri dish full of disease that is not reacting to penicillin. He is going to say something insightful or surprising. I can feel it coming.

"I'd sure appreciate it if you'd take me home," he says flatly, and then turns away.

I stare at the wind chime and swallow hard. He didn't actually ask me to take him home, which he knows I can't do. He made a statement that requires no action, but yet made his feelings known.

I fantasize about taking him home—maybe to the farm in Virginia. I could try to buy it back from the Barbers. He would know exactly where he was there.

Or to Clark Air Base in the Philippines. We could get an apartment and go see the South Seas. He could die where he saved people from dying, instead of dying with patients, Alzheimer's taunting him to the bitter end.

Or, I suppose, I could kill him, which was his original request. That is going home too. Going home to his mother. God, Buddha, Allah and Shiva know that I wanted to kill him many times in my youth when Dr. Bercaw didn't pay any attention to me—or whenever he did, to chastise or frighten or abandon me.

I could easily get my hands on enough meds to end his life. In fact, I could put my entire bottle of antidepressants down his throat. I could plead temporary insanity—or abuse, although all Beau ever did was love me in his own way.

One of my best friends is now a clinical psychologist. She recently told me that I am counterphobic: I prefer fearful situations because my father scared me so much in my youth. Ever since, she says, I seek out what frightens me in an effort to gain control of the fear. This would make a good argument in court. My defense could be counterphobia. My father scared me so much that I was afraid *not* to kill him.

"Bercaws and Filipinos aren't cowards," he told me once.

"Are Filipinos scared of Bercaws?" I responded.

"Everyone's afraid of Bercaws," he answered.

But I have since learned that Bercaws and Filipinos are scared of the same thing: ghosts of the past, and headless ones in particular.

Nora recently said that Beau has a safe-deposit box for me. Over the years, he has filled it with treasures—raw uncut diamonds, rubies and sapphires. Jewels fit for a mermaid's chest.

I can feel our fairy tale coming to an end.

When he is gone, I may take Beau's brain in a jar to Clark Air Base and set it free in the South Seas—to float in salt water, instead of formaldehyde like his father's, no longer trapped by history and fear.

I take out my iPhone and open up the photo album. I show Beau how to scroll through the pictures of my family in Cambodia. He pauses at one of David in front of Angkor Wat and nods.

"Is that your boy?" he asks.

"Yes. That's David Beauregard."

I show him one of Allan, and he looks perplexed. I remember a funny conversation we had fourteen years ago, after he first met Allan.

"Can you believe how happy he is?" I asked my dad.

Beau twisted up his face. "How can you stand it, Gal?"

We laughed.

"Remember when I thought I'd marry Gunther Gebel-Williams from the Ringling Bros. and Barnum & Bailey Circus?"

"Yup, but I thought you'd fall for a big-game hunter in Kenya."

"When I met a Turkish man in Tanzania, you told me that if I couldn't be his first wife, I should be his best wife."

A few years later, over dinner, my father turned to Allan, my first and only husband, and said, "Thank you for making my daughter so happy."

Beau took about 1,100 pictures of us that evening. It was the last time I remember him using his camera. I told my dad that Allan represented the four kinds of love to me. *Eros. Agape. Storge. Philia.* Beau nodded in approval.

Now Beau is enjoying the marvel that is the iPhone. He is going from one picture to the next, and the next, getting faster and faster until he's not really looking at the pictures, just enjoying the scrolling process. The blur itself is pleasing.

Beau pauses on a picture of a car.

"Is that your car?"

"Yes, but there's no gun in the glove box; no gold coins in the trunk."

"You should get some gold coins. The dollar will be worthless one day."

He hands back the iPhone.

"Dad, what's 174 x 20?"

Beau furrows his brow.

"Well, let's see. Four times zero. Hmm. It's 3,480."

I check his math on my iPhone's calculator. He is right. He remembers numbers better than his family. Maybe some of his tactics worked after all. No one else at Juniper can remember anything.

I had called Uncle Pete a month earlier and told him that his brother Beau had Alzheimer's and was in a memory care facility in Naples. Pete lived just a half-hour north in Ft. Myers. He went to visit, but Beau had no idea who Pete was. Beau hadn't seen him since their mother's funeral nine years earlier.

Woodson still lives in his nursing home in Colorado. His mind is intact on some days, and gone on others, but his body is failing fast. My cousin Nancy says that he vacillates between thinking he is the prisoner or the guard at his nursing home.

My dad and I go back to staring at the wind chime. Another resident comes by and sits down on the other side of Beau. Her name is Helen. She has lost the ability to speak clearly. She tries to talk with us. I can't understand a word she says. Beau looks over at her, and cocks his head. He can't make it out either. Twenty years ago, if she had been his patient, or someone like Bruce at Grandmother's nursing home, Beau would have known exactly what she was trying to communicate. I push a tear out of my eye before my father can see it.

"Getting 'bout time for lunch," I say.

Every Thanksgiving of my youth, Beau ordered 100 Virginia hams. When they arrived, I earned extra money by hand-delivering them to all his friends and colleagues, including the radiologists and the

Board of Trustees at Naples Community Hospital. The antitrust case was settled after five years in favor of the hospital, although the court saw merit in Beau's case, and commended him. And as mad as the radiologists and the trustees were, they respected Beau. He fought like a warrior and accepted defeat like a gentleman.

An Asian Virginian.

The only one of his kind, besides me.

After every Thanksgiving dinner, Beau made us walk around the block so that we wouldn't have a stroke. In his years on call at the ER, he had learned that two hours after the standard Thanksgiving dinner mealtime, the phone would ring. He would be called in to attend to a stroke victim, who had lain down after eating a huge meal.

Beau looks at his watch.

"Guess so," he says.

"What do they serve?"

"I don't know, but it gives me diarrhea."

I help him up and take his hand. We walk past the hibisci and some birdhouses from which a few squirrels are pilfering seed.

"Sure is a nice day," I say.

"Especially when that breeze hits," he answers, swinging his hand, which is firmly attached to mine.

POSTSCRIPT

I am in the mountains of Vermont on a farm. I have come here to rest my mind after Beau's death. It is raining outside my cabin now. Oh, how I love the sound of water.

Funny that I chose to retreat into hills instead of seas.

Funny this, too: I went swimming yesterday and the water made me seasick.

As Beau lay dying, I read him the first chapter of this book in which he taught me to swim in Huntsville. I also read portions of *The Little Mermaid* to him. His breathing was labored. His left arm was curled up around his neck like a python. His face was gaunt. His limbs were whiter than white. He had apnea, and I wondered if I should give him a tracheotomy. I wanted him back. Every second of every minute of my life with him.

Clark. Garuda. Virginia. Gators. Kenya. Jeeps. Rebelanna. Vans. Books. Rivers. Pools. Books. Oreos. Snickers Bars. Beans. Angkor. Communists. Capitalists. Tree houses. Battlegrounds. Brains in jars.

But with my father's last breath, at 6:30 a.m. on April 2, 2012, our story ended.

EPILOGUE

Dear David,

When we returned from Singapore, in the summer of 2010, we had lunch with Grandpa Beau at the Perkins Restaurant in Naples. You were fidgety and loud, as any six-year-old would be. Beau, who was slipping fast but still fairly alert, stared at you the entire time.

I asked Beau who you were acting like, fully expecting him to look at me and say, "You, Gal."

Instead, he pointed to himself.

David, when you read this book, and come to understand your mother and our family, I want you to know that you are not Beau and neither am I. We may have some of his genes, but we are free to make our own choices in our lives and not be gripped and paralyzed by things that may or may not happen to us.

You are nearly nine and I'm nearly forty-seven. I don't want to spend the second half of my time on Earth worrying about whether or not I'm going to get

Alzheimer's disease. I'd rather show you the world than take supplements or do long math. I'm choosing my father's love of adventure to pass down to you rather than his fear of losing his mind.

Beau once asked me to write a book with him about how to stave off "what his father had" through his well-researched protocol. I refused as politely as I could. I knew his protocol wasn't going to work. I think he did too. Alzheimer's disease defined him. There was no escaping it. To him, Bercaws and Alzheimer's were part of the same double helix. But he neglected—or perhaps conveniently forgot—that we have some control over who we become.

This is who I am: a swimmer and writer driven by my own decisions and composition. I am happiest setting foot on new territory even if it feels like I'm walking on knives, like the Little Mermaid. Unknowingly, Beau spent his lifetime preparing me for suffering. It's what he felt he had to do.

And this is what I had to do: Write a book about a doctor so fixated on losing his memory that it drove him to the brink of sanity; and, his Gal, who learned to swim in a sea of ambiguity. It seemed to me that writing about my life with Beau might be more instructional than a manual of how to take brain-saving supplements. The deep and terrible irony is that Beau lost many opportunities to make more memories because he was consumed with saving the ones he'd already accumulated. In the end, he remembered math better than his family.

When I visited Beau the February before he died, he looked at me long and hard. I sat down next to him. He stared right at me—or through me. I knew something crazy was forthcoming. He had that look. Typically he didn't smile, though, when he was about to make a pronouncement, like when he asked me to kill him if he turned out like his father.

But Beau's eyes were lit up and a big grin overtook his face. Does he remember me? Does he recall camping or canoeing? Does he love me?

I waited.

Beau giggled and then, very purposely and slowly said, "Funny how things turn out." I laughed with him.

Through a haze of tangled plaque, Dr. Beauregard Lee Bercaw suddenly saw his life with perfect clarity.

So let me be clear with you, my son. If I do get Alzheimer's disease, it's okay. We'll have so many memories by then that we won't be able to remember them all anyway. Forgetting my life won't change my love for you.

When you and I rode the bus to your school in Singapore every day, no one around us spoke English. There was Mandarin, Hindi and Arabic. I didn't understand a thing that was being said. I liked it! I realized then and there that you don't have to comprehend everything. At that moment, on that public bus in Asia, I accepted my father for the person he was. I stopped trying to figure him out. And, thereby, set myself free. I realized, too, that I felt closest to my father when I was in places he loved instead of by his side.

Memories fade. Will my life grow more worthless with each blurred recollection? Not a chance. Life is measured in love—not brain mass. I struggle to remember my dead stepbrother's face now, but I still love Craig as much as I ever did. And I certainly don't remember the Philippines of my youth, but I adore it just the same. Feeling trumps thinking. Remember that.

I want you to go live your own life. As for me, if genetics repeats itself, it'll be like that bus in Singapore. I don't need to know what's happening to be content. When all is said and done, I hope you will discover what Beau never did in all his searching.

It's the heart that belongs in a jar.

Love,
Your Mother

ACKNOWLEDGMENTS

I can't thank my husband Allan Nicholls enough. He found all the old letters and photos included in this book—all of which my Uncle Woodson had given me after Grandmother died. Allan also patiently waited while my mind fixated on my father's mind for more than two years.

I also am grateful to my son David Beauregard Nicholls for listening to these stories and deciding which ones were "good."

I thank my father Beauregard Lee Bercaw for the adventure of a lifetime. I love you, ol' dad. And, yes, I am a buzzard tail, as these pages attest.

I have to offer my deep gratitude to former U.S. Senator Bob Kerrey and former U.S. Speaker of the House Newt Gingrich for writing such a beautiful and compelling introduction. I love the serendipity of their contribution: Bob, the Democrat, as my friend; and Newt, the Republican, as Beau's hero. They represent us so very well indeed: a tension of opposites within the very same system.

Thanks to Robert Egge, Vice President of Public Policy and Advocacy for the Alzheimer's Association, for his support and assistance.

I also praise the following family members who inspired and sustained me: my mother Barbara Rixey Darrow; my brother Lee Rixey Bercaw, his wife Kelly and their children Alyssa and Christopher; my stepmother Nora Fairbrother Bercaw, who was so dedicated to my father—and he to her; Trisha Fairbrother Hollowell; my stepsister Kathy Marshall Dion, her husband Paul and their children Hannah and Allison; my deceased stepbrother Craig Richard Marshall and his former wife Leslie; my cousin Nancy Dunlap Bercaw and her brothers Woodson and John; my deceased uncle Woodson Woods Bercaw and his ex-wife Sue Allison; my uncle Peter Bercaw; my deceased uncle David Meade Bercaw and his widow Penny and daughter Kathy; my cousin Pamela Scott Arnold; my uncle Scott Stratton and his wife Kathy, and son Garrett; my stepchildren and their wives, John and Ashley Nicholls and Andrew and Samantha Nicholls.

Also, many thanks to Kent and Harriet Loving, for looking after Bercaw affairs for far too long. Thank you, as well, to Lyles Baptist Church, where all Bercaws are blessed and buried.

I could not have written *Brain in a Jar* without the tireless support of the following people and organizations: Kelly Dineen; Margaret Mary King; Maureen King; Nancy and Ned Foster; Pamela Polston of *Seven Days* newspaper; David Corcoran and Mike Mason of the *New York Times*; Mara Saule and the Libraries at the University of Vermont; Carol Capitani; Deb Lichtenfeld; Tracy Treadwell; Jess Oski; Aimee Petrin; C.D. Mattison; Jill McManus; Jon Shenton; Stephen Figueroa; Ken Heilman, M.D., and the University of Florida Brain Institute; Charles Anderson, M.D.; Matt Baker, M.D.; Andy Lipman, M.D.; Mike Lusk, M.D.; Steve DeKosky, M.D., and the University of Virginia Medical School; John Eagle, M.D.; Eric Reiman, M.D., of the Banner Alzheimer's Institute; Francisco Lopera, M.D., and Yakeel T. Quiroz, Ph.D., of Universidad de Antioquia; Brooke Barss, M.D.; Christine Staats, M.D.; Frank Williams, M.D. and Jackie Williams; Selene Colburn; Peter Spitzform; Margot Harrison; Angela and Greg Collins; Joe Dineen and Claudia Case Scarfone; Mike and Pat Dalton; Al and Judy Justice; Coach Dick Smith and Carlouel Yacht Club; the swim teams at the University of Vermont, New York University, and James Madison University;

the athletic department at the University of South Florida; Professor Lawrence Broer; the perfection and grace that is Kathryn Altman; Haley DuMond and her father Don; Keith Carradine; Kansas Carradine; Sandra and Marcia Langley; Bill and Tyler Stafford; Samantha Hunt; Thomas Gustafson; the staff at Juniper Village in Naples; Vanessa and Blanche Hansen; Tommy Hansen; Wayne and Barbara Grigsby; Kris Nicholls; Monica Lowy; Christine Sigman; Jen Kircher; Philip Baruth; Erik Esckilsen; Nora Jacobsen and David Ferm; Naples Community Hospital; Rich and Nancy Kirchner of First United Method Church of Naples; Robin Lauzon Parker; Darren Higgins; Michael Mann; Sky Meadow Retreat; Jane and Terry Smith; Tom and Lynn Brennan; Heather Eves; Pamela O'-Callaghan; Scott Cory; Karen Jean Hunt; John Tierney; Lisa Kusel; Veronica Bulgari; Barbara Becker; Peter Blackmer; Ung Savy; Liz Jensen; Liesel Duhon; Jamie Amelio; Angie Jackson; Nancy Zuccaro; Martha Richardson and the Vermont Alzheimer's Association; the very special Merit Greaves; and, all the Rixeys whom I love dearly. And special thanks to Sam Rixey for designing my website.

Very, very special thanks to my agents Priya Doraswamy and Jayapriya Vasudevan. And, finally, I have gratitude galore for Larry W. Moore, Sheila Bucy Potter, Stephan Taylor, and Jonathan Greene of Broadstone Books because, by publishing *Brain in a Jar*, they have ensured that my father's memory will always be alive and well.